Amputation, Prosthesis Use, and Phantom Limb Pain

Craig Murray
Editor

Amputation, Prosthesis Use, and Phantom Limb Pain

An Interdisciplinary Perspective

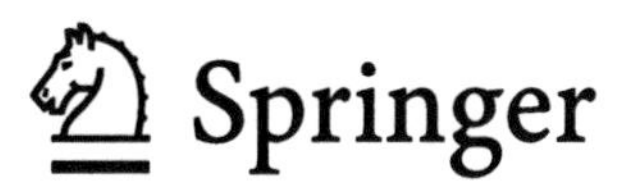

Editor
Craig Murray
School of Health & Medicine
Division of Health Research, Bowland Tower East
Lancaster University
Lancaster LA1 4YT, UK
c.murray@lancaster.ac.uk

ISBN 978-0-387-87461-6 e-ISBN 978-0-387-87462-3
DOI 10.1007/978-0-387-87462-3
Springer New York Dordrecht Heidelberg London

Library of Congress Control Number: 2009939836

Printed on acid-free paper

Springer is part of Springer Science+Business Media (www.springer.com)

Contents

Contributors

Dr. Elaine Biddiss is a researcher at the Bloorview Research Institute, University of Toronto, Canada. Her research interests include wearable sensors and actuators; user-centered, context aware interfaces; and multi-modal feedback. She has published widely on prosthesis use, including on consumer design priorities for prostheses.

Helena Burger is a researcher at the Institute of Rehabilitation, Ljubljana, Slovenia. She has published extensively on amputation and prosthesis use, including the topics of service provision and evaluation of prosthesis use.

Dr. Deirdre Desmond is a Lecturer in Psychology in the Department of Psychology at the National University of Ireland Maynooth and co-director of the Dublin Psychoprosthetics Group. Her interest in psychosocial adjustment to amputation and prosthesis use stems from her doctoral work which was completed at Trinity College Dublin in collaboration with the British Limbless Ex-Service Men's Association. Dr. Desmond is currently serving as an Associate Editor with *Prosthetics and Orthotics International*, the official journal of the International Society for Prosthetics and Orthotics (ISPO).

Dr. Pamela Gallagher is a Senior Lecturer in Psychology in the Faculty of Science and Health, School of Nursing, Dublin City University, Ireland. She co-directs the Dublin Psychoprosthetics Group (www.tcd.ie/psychoprosthetics): a unique multi-disciplinary group of international researchers and clinicians interested in applying many and varied aspects of psychology to prosthetic use.

Dr. Kate Grady is a Consultant in Anaesthesia & Pain Medicine at University Hospital of South Manchester, UK.

Toby Howard is a Senior Lecturer in the School of Computer Science at The University of Manchester, UK, and a founder member of the Advanced Interfaces Group. His research interests include applications of virtual environments to interdisciplinary research such as psychology, and to real-world problems, with particular application to scene-of-crime reconstruction and forensic analysis. He also works on non-photorealistic computer graphics, and is enthusiastic about academic outreach and public understanding of science.

Laurence Kenney is a Senior Research Fellow with the Centre for Rehabilitation and Human Performance Research at the University of Salford, UK. His research focuses on the development and evaluation of rehabilitation technologies, particularly prosthetics and functional electrical-stimulation systems. He received his PhD in engineering design from the University of Salford and is a member of the Institute of Physics and Engineering in Medicine. He has recently been appointed Associate Editor for *Prosthetics and Orthotics International.*

Dr. Jai Kulkarni, MA, FRCP, is a Consultant and Honorary Reader in Rehabilitation Medicine at the University Hospital of South Manchester, UK. His main interests are amputee rehabilitation and neurological rehabilitation. In the field of amputee rehabilitation his active interests are in falls, post-amputation pain management, post-amputation arthritis and congenital limb deficiencies. He has co-authored a succinct white coat pocket book on prescribing upper limb prosthesis and has close links with both the University of Salford and the University of Manchester.

Dr. Donna Lloyd is a Lecturer in Psychology at the University of Manchester, UK. Her main research interests are the mechanisms underlying sensory processing, body perception and spatial awareness in healthy and clinical populations using cognitive neuroscience techniques including functional magnetic resonance imaging (fMRI). More recently, her work has explored the behavioural and neural mechanisms underlying phantom sensations and illusory sensations of touch. Her recent papers include "Phantom limb pain, cortical reorganisation and the therapeutic effect of mental imagery" (*Brain*, 2009), and "Development of a paradigm for measuring somatic disturbance in clinical populations with medically unexplained symptoms" (*Journal of Psychosomatic Research*, 2008).

Kate MacIver has worked in pain management for the past 13 years – for the past 4 years as a Research Fellow at the Pain Research Institute in Liverpool, UK, and prior to that as a Clinical Nurse Specialist in pain management at the Walton Centre for Neurology and Neurosurgery also in Liverpool. Her research interests include quantitative sensory testing and mechanisms of neuropathic pain; phantom limb pain; central pain in multiple sclerosis and spinal cord injury.

Professor Mac MacLachlan is an Associate Professor in the School of Psychology and Centre for Global Health, Trinity College Dublin. His research interests are in psychoprosthetics and disability, culture and health, and organisational aspects of international aid. Much of his research is currently based in Africa. He is Extraordinary Professor of Disability and Development, at the Centre for Rehabilitation Studies, Stellenbosch University, South Africa; and Research Advisor to the Southern African Federation of the Disabled. Mac has a longstanding interest in disability spanning voluntary work, practice as a clinical psychologist, consultancy and as a researcher and lecturer.

Dr. Craig Murray is a Senior Lecturer in Psychology in the Institute of Health Research at Lancaster University, UK. He is particularly interested in embodiment and mental health and has been involved in a number of projects surrounding amputation, prosthesis use and phantom limb pain for the past 15 years. He is editor of the *Psychological Scientific Perspectives on Out-of-Body Experiences* (2009 Nova Science Publishers, New York).

Joanne Murray is a Research Associate at the Institute of Health Research, Lancaster University, UK.

Emma Patchick is a Research Associate in the School of Psychological Sciences at the University of Manchester, UK.

Dr. Steve Pettifer is a Senior Lecturer in The School of Computer Science at The University of Manchester, UK, and a member of the Advanced Interfaces Group. His research interests include virtual environments, scientific visualisation, distributed computing and human computer interaction. Much of his current research revolves around making data in the life sciences comprehensible through interactive visualisation techniques.

Elisabeth Schaffalitzky is a Research Student in the School of Nursing, Dublin City University, Ireland.

Mohammad Sobuh received the BSc degree in Orthotics and Prosthetics from the University of Jordan in 2004, and his MSc by research degree in upper limb prostheses from Salford University in 2008, and is currently carrying out his PhD in upper limb prostheses, also at Salford, UK. His MSc research has focused on upper limb prosthetic evaluation and activity monitoring. His research interests include upper limb prosthetic kinematics, upper limb prosthetic evaluation and activity monitoring.

Cliff Richardson, BSc (Hons), RGN, MSc, PhD, is a Lecturer in Adult Nursing at the University of Manchester, UK. His nursing career (London, Manchester, Bolton) was mainly focussed on the care of surgical patients. In 1993 he set up and ran an acute pain service. In 1999 he took up a fellowship at Liverpool John Moores University and the Pain Research Institute where he completed his PhD on phantom limb pain. He moved to Manchester University in 2004.

Dr. Martin Twiste is a Senior Lecturer at the University of Salford, UK, within the Directorate of Prosthetics & Orthotics. His research focuses on upper and lower limb prostheses with particular emphasis on motion analysis, quantifying prosthetic component behaviour, and designing improved prosthetic components. Recent studies investigated the effects of lateral whip gait deviations, of a self-aligning prosthetic foot, of alignment changes, and of prosthesis properties on amputee gait, as well as the characteristics of upper limb prosthetic movement in reaching and grasping, and the relationship between socket design and low levels of usage and functionality in myoelectric prostheses.

Chapter 1
Developing an Interdisciplinary Perspective on Amputation, Prosthesis Use, and Phantom Limb Pain: An Introduction

Craig Murray

The impetus for the current book developed from the establishment of the *Interdisciplinary Prosthetics Research Network* in the United Kingdom, which held a conference to develop the book in June 2008. The aim of the conference was to encourage dialogue between the range of professionals and disciplines engaged in research and practice related to limb loss and prosthesis use. To this end, the Network and contributors to the book include biomedical engineers, computer scientists, nurses, prosthetists, psychologists, neuroscientists, and rehabilitation consultants, along with world-renowned research groups that have specialisms in the themes of the book (for example the Advanced Interfaces Group at the University of Manchester, the Pain Research Institute at Liverpool University, and the Centre for Rehabilitation and Human Performance Research at the University of Salford). In addition, the group has a wide range of multi-disciplinary, world-wide research collaborators, some of whom have made chapter contributions here.

The book focuses on the related topics of amputation, prosthesis use and phantom limb pain, written by contributors who are leading researchers in their field. It comprises three broad inter-related sections, which together elucidate key developments and thinking within these topic areas. Following this introductory chapter in which the topics and chapters of the book are overviewed, the first section concentrates on the work of prosthetists and biomedical engineers and comprises three chapters. Together these chapters explicate the processes involved in prosthetists' work with clients in a manner which will be of interest to students and professionals from a range of disciplines.

In the first of these, Elaine Biddiss, a biomedical engineer, argues that user-centred design is essential to the development of prostheses that better meet consumer needs. Consideration of this leads to priorities directed towards improving comfort (e.g., by reducing the weight of current devices), life-like function and appearance, and enhanced sensory feedback. Biddiss discusses how prosthesis

---

C. Murray
School of Health and Medicine, Division of Health Research, Bowland Tower East, Lancaster University, Lancaster, LA1 4YT, UK
e-mail: c.murray@lancaster.ac.uk

C. Murray (ed.), *Amputation, Prosthesis Use, and Phantom Limb Pain: An Interdisciplinary Perspective*, DOI 10.1007/978-0-387-87462-3_1,

acceptance and quality of life can be increased with reduced costs and more efficient funding for prostheses and healthcare services, better access to repairs and maintenance, and by having multiple and activity-specific prostheses. She also suggests that prosthesis acceptance rates and consumer satisfaction can be improved with timely fitting and by involving consumers actively in the selection of their prosthesis.

Next, Jai Kulkarni, a clinician responsible for the provision of prosthetics in a large regional area of the UK, presents a range of ethical and medico-legal issues for rehabilitation professionals in the supply and withdrawal of prostheses and assistive technology for people with limb loss or deformity. He argues that the primary duty of the clinician is to act in the best interests of the patient. However, until recently the ethical considerations involved in amputee prosthetic rehabilitation have not been fully reflected upon. The ethical principles of relevance here include respect for autonomy, non-maleficence, beneficence and justice. Kulkarni outlines how ethical dilemmas arise in relation to goal setting, patient selection, resource allocation, teamwork issues and the expectations of patients. In considering these issues as they arise in the UK, Kulkarni notes there is an element of rationing in health service provision due to lack of resources and doctors are pushed into the role of gatekeepers. The issues discussed here are not particular to the UK, indeed Kulkarni suggests that these issues are common concerns for different countries and settings, even when the practical mechanisms by which service provision is implemented differ.

In the final chapter in this section, members of the Centre for Rehabilitation and Human Performance Research at the University of Salford present the development of an innovative computerised technique for monitoring upper limb prosthesis activity. These researchers argue that the traditional methods for evaluating the functionality provided by upper limb prostheses lack sufficient validity. In response, they report on the development of technology to classify upper limb activities using an artificial neural network as a first step towards the development of an accelerometer-based activity monitor for prosthetic evaluation. Presenting their empirical data on this, the authors suggest that movement patterns of upper limbs in amputees associated with a particular tightly-defined set of tasks are sufficiently characteristic to be distinguished from each other using a neural network. They conclude by discussing further work needed to explore the performance of the classifier in a less constrained environment as a requirement before a definite conclusion can be drawn as to the viability of such an approach.

The next section of the book focuses on psychological and practical aspects of amputation, limb deficiency and prosthesis use. The first of four chapters, written by members of the Dublin Psychoprosthetics Group, explores the ways in which people adapt and cope with limb loss and using a prosthesis, the potential for positive adjustment and strengths emerging from the experience, pain, affective distress, issues around identity, body image and the construction of self and quality of life. It also considers the importance of these issues for health service providers across the multi-disciplinary team who work with people with limb loss. The authors conclude that the ways in which people respond to amputation and prosthesis use are both complex and individual. However, they suggest that consideration of psycho-social factors across the continuum of care can serve to support positive adaptation and to improve outcomes and service delivery.

The second chapter in this section by Craig Murray, a qualitative researcher in health and clinical psychology, expands upon these issues by considering how an understanding of adjustment and coping can be achieved through a consideration of the lived experience of limb loss or absence and prosthesis use. Drawing upon a large-scale qualitative research study, Murray argues that examining the meanings and experience of illness and disability from the vantage point of those concerned enables a better understanding of what it is to cope or adapt, and how this is negotiated. He argues that conceptualisation and theory of coping and adaptation can be usefully informed by the perspectives of those having the relevant experience rather than through the application of a priori theoretical frameworks. Such an approach highlights the subtle and complex ways in which such persons manage, negotiate and experience their identity in everyday life, and therefore how they adapt and cope to their changing circumstances. He concludes by discussing how the outcomes of this work have a number of implications for health professionals working with this client group.

The third and fourth chapters of this section expand upon two key areas that are implicated in the adaptation and coping of persons to limb loss, limb absence and prosthesis use. First, Helena Burger discusses returning to work following amputation, which she argues is one aspect of the rehabilitative aim to restore or improve functioning following limb loss. However, such persons frequently experience problems returning to work, and may need to change occupation as a result of their limb loss. Such post-amputation jobs are generally physically less demanding, but are more complex with a requirement for a higher level of general educational attainment. Burger presents a range of factors implicated in the return to work, including age, gender and educational level; as well as factors related to impairments and disabilities due to amputation. She concludes by arguing that vocational rehabilitation and counselling should become a part of rehabilitation programs for all persons following amputation who are of working age, and that better cooperation between professionals and employers is necessary. Following this, Craig Murray discusses the relationships between gender, sexuality and prosthesis use, and the implications of these for rehabilitation. Besides overviewing key literature on sexual functioning and concerns following limb loss, Murray also highlights shortcomings of such research. In particular, he highlights how current research overlooks how sexual concerns may change over time, and how responses to limb losses are likely to be gendered experiences. He reports findings from a qualitative project on the complementary issues of gender, sexuality and romantic relationships, and brings to light how issues of sexuality emerge in relation to other salient meanings and experiences. In contrast to prior research which has had a tendency to explore sexual function and concerns in isolation, Murray's analysis highlights these as gendered concerns and related to issues of forming romantic, as well as sexual, relationships. Murray argues that these findings add support to calls to facilitate discussion about sexuality in the rehabilitation process to aid alleviation of patients' sexuality-based anxieties which, in turn, can help to improve their quality of life.

The final section focuses on pain in the residual limb or stump, phantom limb pain, and emerging treatments and therapies for such conditions. The first of four chapters, by Jai Kulkarni and Kate Grady, presents a clinician's account of post-amputation pain, stressing how this is temporally dependent, varying at different stages of the peri-operative/postoperative period, with possibly more than one pain being present at any time. In considering the complex amalgam of pain contributors, the authors argue for a full biopsychosocial assessment to be made with attention and treatment given to any associated mood disorder, disorder of cognition or behavioural maladaptations. These considerations are developed further in the following two chapters. In the first, written by Cliff Richardson, the literature regarding phantom limb pain (PLP) following limb amputation is reviewed. Richardson notes that controversies exist over the incidence and prevalence, causes, mechanisms and management of phantom limb pain. He argues that to ensure rigour, before addressing factors that are associated with PLP, it is necessary to tackle controversies within PLP. To this end, he reviews each area of controversy and concludes with consideration of what appear to be aspects of the individual that play a role in PLP development and/or maintenance.

Following this Kate MacIver and Donna Lloyd provide a comprehensive overview of the management of chronic PLP as it relates to the patient in the prosthesis clinic. The chapter begins with phantom pain assessment and discusses the efficacy, side effects and advice that needs to be given to patients regarding pharmacological therapies before presenting psychological aspects of treatment. These include how to recognise psychological distress; how to know when to refer on for psychological treatment, and promising psychological interventions. The chapter concludes with suggestions for the holistic management of patients suffering from PLP.

The final chapter in this section is written by members of the Advanced Interfaces Group at the University of Manchester, who present virtual reality (VR) as an emerging therapy for PLP. Current applications involve movements of an alternative or the remaining portion of an anatomical limb to control a virtual or 'phantom' limb, The authors note that the use of this technology emerges from work using a mirror box, where the reflection of an intact limb into the phenomenal space of the absent has been found to evoke kinaesthetic sensations in the phantom limb and in some cases reduce PLP. This development had been driven by both the promise of mirror box work and its inherent limitations with regards to its flexibility in providing a fully robust illusion of an absent limb as intact. The authors present the practical implementation and empirical work arising from their own immersive virtual reality system alongside those of two other research groups (those of the Dublin Psychoprosthetics Group and Jonathan Cole's group). They argue that although further work is needed (most notably controlled, large-scale quantitative evaluations), there are promising lines of findings from these interrelated strands of research that are suggestive of the potential for VR to provide effective relief for PLP.

Taken together, the chapters in the current volume make a significant contribution to the interrelated topics of amputation, prosthesis use and phantom limb pain, and demonstrate how professionals from a variety of backgrounds can benefit from creating a dialogue with one another in order to better address these topics. It is hoped that this collection serves as a valuable resource for students, researchers and practitioners. It is also hoped that it will help to further stimulate the cross-fertilisation of research ideas among the different disciplines represented herein. If so, this will undoubtedly lead not only to an increase in knowledge about these topics, but to improvements in service provision and care for the client group around whom the authors' contributions revolve.

Chapter 2
Need-Directed Design of Prostheses and Enabling Resources

Elaine Biddiss

Abstract In this chapter, we address questions of prosthesis acceptance, design, and supporting resources from the perspective of consumer needs. Throughout, the observations presented are largely based on the experiences of approximately 250 individuals with upper limb absence, and are supported by the literature of the past 25 years. The choice to accept or reject a prosthesis is largely dictated by personal needs and is made in such a way so as to optimize quality of life. Prosthesis design should first focus on maximizing comfort, particularly by reducing the weight and improving the thermal properties of current models. Consumers are also interested in reduced costs, enhanced sensory feedback, and life-like dexterity and appearance. Ongoing initiatives and technological development to address these consumer design priorities are discussed. Lastly, perspectives on enabling healthcare and economic resources fundamental to the prescription and availability of prostheses are outlined. Clinical strategies to promote prosthesis acceptance are identified and consumer-directed recommendations for social support structures are detailed.

2.1 Introduction

> "This coming January will be the 40 year anniversary of my LBE (left limb, below elbow) amputation. I feel truly blessed with what I've been able to do with my body powered prosthesis and the fact that it has enabled me to do everything I've set out to do. I honestly feel the only opportunities that have been closed to me have been the result of others' limited understanding. Since my amputation, I've become a Commercial/Instrument Pilot, and Expert, D-Licensed Skydiver and have enjoyed an excellent business career that has taken me to President and Director. I'd have to say, the limb loss has not been a deterrent at all. And, maybe, in some situations, it has actually been a help. Prostheses have been a challenge from time to time because of limited access to facilities and repair/maintenance issues. However, with each repair, we've been able to increase strength and some function. So now, it's pretty solid and the fact that I always have a back-up system to change into, makes any repair almost a non-event."

E. Biddiss
Bloorview Research Institute, Bloorview Kids Rehab, Totonto ON Canada, Institute of Biometerials and Biomedical Engineering, University of Toronto, Toronto, ON, Canada
e-mail: elaine.biddiss@utoronto.ca

C. Murray (ed.), *Amputation, Prosthesis Use, and Phantom Limb Pain: An Interdisciplinary Perspective*, DOI 10.1007/978-0-387-87462-3_2,

- "Jack", 64 years

"In our experience, we found nothing our daughter could do with the prosthesis that she couldn't already do better, faster or more efficiently without it. We were so excited about the opportunity to try the technology but it was immediately obvious that it didn't improve her quality of life, particularly at her young age. It was frustrating, hot, heavy and she had to LEARN to do things with it that she already did very well with her natural arm. It just wasn't necessary. This does not mean we wouldn't give something new and different a try as technology advanced. It just wasn't right at the time, and hasn't been again since."

- Mother of "Sarah", 8 years

Sarah and Jack are two unique individuals, with different likes and dislikes, different lifestyles, and different experiences with limb absence. Each has made the personal choice to use or not use prostheses in a way that optimizes their own quality of life. Both are happy in their choice and are confident, enthusiastic people. In the case of Sarah and Jack, access to resources has not been a factor in their decisions and their choices are motivated strictly by their own personal attributes and needs. This is not always the case. The mission of policy makers, healthcare practitioners, and prosthesis designers is to ensure that the best possible resources are made available to each individual, empowering them with choices that enable them to achieve their personal goals. In this chapter, we discuss user perspectives on the quality and availability of these resources. We identify factors motivating prosthesis use or non-use. Lastly, we detail specific recommendations for the prescription, design, and funding of upper limb prostheses to better meet consumer needs.

The insights reflected in this chapter are grounded in literature of the past 25 years enhanced by the wide breadth of experience of approximately 250 individuals garnered from an international survey on upper limb absence (Biddiss et al. 2007; Biddiss and Chau 2007a; Biddiss and Chau 2008a). A snapshot of their demographic distribution is presented in Table 2.1. The interested reader is referred to the following for methodological details pertaining to this survey (Biddiss et al. 2007; Biddiss and Chau 2007a; Biddiss and Chau 2008a).

2.2 Prosthesis Acceptance: A Question of Need

If a person feels that a prosthesis enhances their function and/or appearance, they will use the device. Conversely, if the prosthesis is perceived to hinder function or comfort, or spoil appearance, they will not use the device. Simple though they may be, these two corollaries succinctly capture the motivations behind prosthesis use or abandonment. The two most commonly reported reasons for non-use are (Biddiss and Chau 2007) (a) Just as or more functional without it (reported by 98% of non-wearers), and (b) More comfortable without it (95% of non-wearers). More interesting is the question: What makes a prosthesis useful to one person, and not useful to or suitable for the next?

Prosthesis technology is optimally designed for the most prevalent trans-radial limb absence and this is reflected in prosthesis acceptance rates (Biddiss and Chau 2007a, b). At lower levels of limb absence, fitting may be increasingly difficult given the longer residua.

Table 2.1 Demographics of survey participants

Population characteristics	Participants ($N=242$)
Levels of Limb absence	16%
Distal to wrist	54%
Trans-radial	21%
Trans-humeral	7%
Proximal to shoulder	
Bilateral limb absence	15%
Origin of limb absence	58%
Congenital	42%
Acquired	
Gender	51%
Male	49%
Female	
Age	43 ± 15 years, 19–80 years
Adults ($N=145$)	9.5 ± 6 years, 1–18 years
Pediatric ($N=97$)	
Country	35%
Canada	43%
United States	17%
Europe	5%
Other	
Follow-upWearers (time since first prosthesis fitting)	17 ± 14 years (0–50 years)
Non-wearers (time since prosthesis rejection)	12 ± 13 years (1–61 years)

Sensory feedback, which is lost when the residual limb is enclosed within the prosthesis, may be more sorely missed; or the individual may simply discover that the long residual limb and/or partial hand are sufficient to perform activities of daily living. At higher levels of limb absence, limitations in prosthesis function (lack of shoulder rotation, complex and discontinuous control schemes) and discomfort (heavy weight, poor fit, lack of heat dissipation) motivate many individuals to adapt to life without a prosthesis. This is particularly true for individuals with congenital limb absence at the higher or lower levels or bilateral limb absence (Biddiss and Chau 2007a). For these individuals, there is and has never been a “sense of arm” and hence, they increasingly find it easier to adapt to their limb differences without the perceived discomfort or functional limitations of prostheses. The opposite may be true particularly for males with acquired limb absence for whom prosthesis acceptance appears to be high (Biddiss and Chau 2007a). Literature exploring factors in technology abandonment strongly supports the role of level of limb absence in prosthesis acceptance (Biddiss and Chau 2007b). Evidence with regards to other factors (e.g., gender, age, etc.) remains contradictory and is likely secondary to level of limb absence. For a detailed review of the literature pertaining to motivations in prosthesis use and acceptance, the interested reader is referred to (Biddiss and Chau 2007b).

Prosthesis rejection and usage rates are widely reported and a review of these is provided in (Biddiss and Chau 2007c). Figure 2.1 presents those associated with the survey presented herein, whereas Fig. 2.2 indicates the acceptance rates of various prosthesis types.

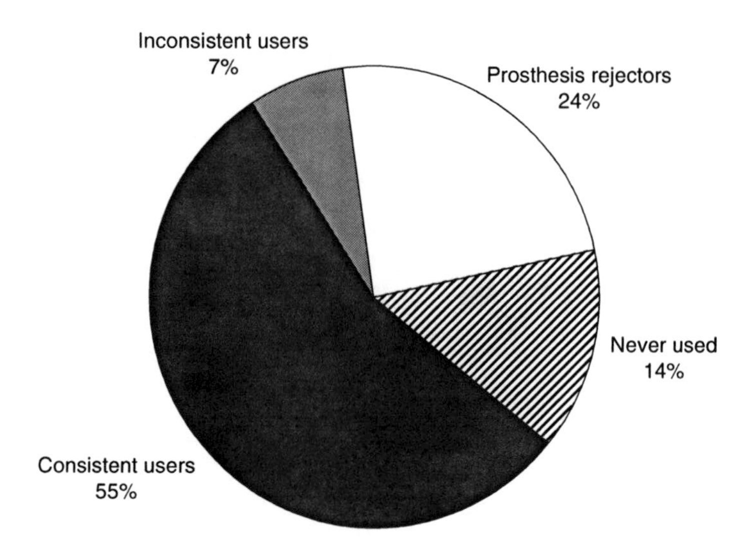

Fig. 2.1 Prosthesis acceptance and usage patterns

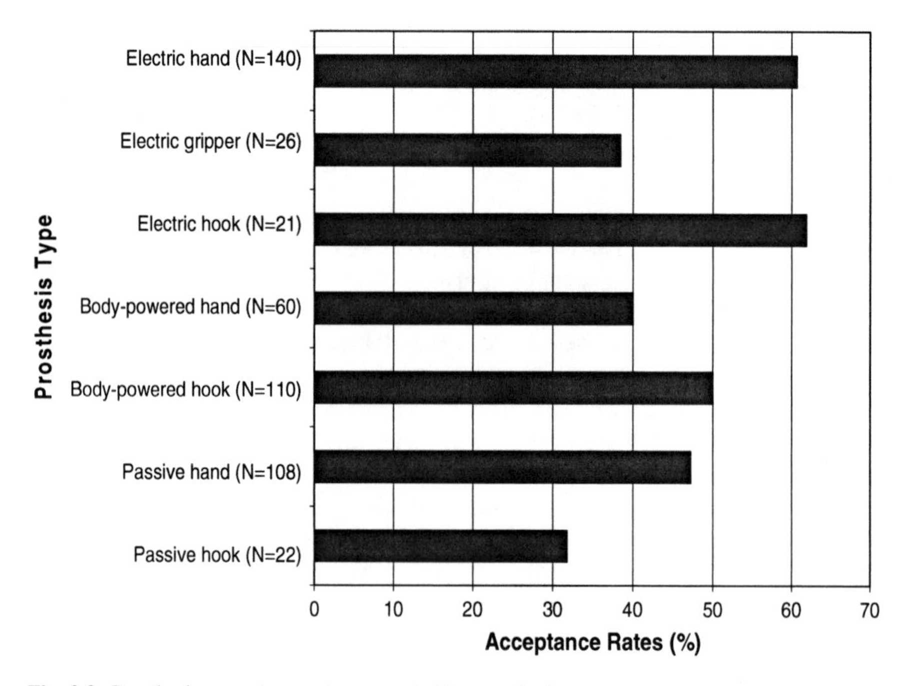

Fig. 2.2 Prosthesis acceptance rates presented by prosthesis type

These values are perhaps lower than the average reported in the literature, although well within the extremely large standard deviations (Biddiss and Chau 2007c). Higher rates of rejection are likely owing to the specific recruitment strategies adopted in this survey, wherein participants were engaged both from community and hospital based networks.

Previous studies have largely focused on the latter and may therefore be biased towards individuals still using prostheses and in contact with these healthcare services. Prosthesis rejection and usage patterns should be regarded with extreme caution. They are highly context-specific and vary largely depending on availability of resources, funding structures, study methodology (e.g., time of follow-up, definition of prosthesis rejection), together with countless characteristics specific to the participants themselves (e.g., level and origin of limb absence). Formulating conclusions pertaining to the innate value of a prosthesis based on rejection rates and usage patterns is not recommended for the following reasons:

1. A person may choose to wear or not to wear a prosthesis and still retain a very high quality of life. However, it does not follow that their quality of life would be equivalent should the opportunity to sample the technology and determine its suitability for their needs be withheld.
2. A device may be used on a part-time or sporadic basis, but still be considered essential for quality of life. For example, an individual may restrict prosthesis use to ensure that it is in good condition for those activities where it is vitally needed. Alternatively, the prosthesis may serve a very specific purpose (e.g., preparing dinner) that may not require full-time use, but would be sorely missed if the prosthesis was not available when required.
3. Personal needs are dynamic and fluctuating. One type of device may suit an individual's needs at one particular life stage, but not at another. For example, passive devices are often prescribed for young children or recent amputees. These individuals may subsequently adopt active prostheses. The passive prosthesis may be defined as a "rejected" technology, however it served a much-needed purpose at a particular time and should therefore be viewed as a successful fitting.

The primary goal of defining rejection and acceptance rates should be to identify groups of individuals whose needs may not be adequately addressed by current prosthetic and healthcare resources, and perhaps to facilitate matching of individuals with the most appropriate technology for their particular needs. From the rejection rates observed in the survey reported herein, two primary groups in need of more focused design efforts and healthcare emerge (a) Individuals with high level limb absence, (b) Individuals with bilateral limb absence. Satisfaction with prostheses and healthcare resources is significantly lower for these particular groups (Biddiss et al. 2007; Biddiss and Chau 2007a).

The choice of prosthesis type is also largely reflective of personal needs. Individuals with high level limb absence are more likely to choose a body-powered hook for comfort and function, as are individuals with bilateral limb absence (Biddiss et al. 2007). Cost is also of great concern to wearers of body-powered prostheses and not surprisingly, use of these devices tends to be higher in countries where funding systems are less supportive of prosthesis procurement and maintenance (Biddiss et al. 2007; Biddiss and Chau 2007a). Individuals selecting a passive device value appearance more highly than those who choose an active prosthesis (Biddiss et al. 2007). Nevertheless, it is important to emphasize that passive prostheses are also functional devices – they are used to stabilize and support objects and also play important roles in self-image and social confidence, key aspects of the overall quality of life.

In social situations, prostheses of all types are often reportedly used to reduce self-consciousness or to alleviate the discomfort of others.

Depending on the person, a prosthesis can represent an embodied and innate extension of their body; for others, a friend or tool, and, for yet others, an alien entity that is viewed with physical and/or psychological discomfort. These perspectives depend largely on the technological and social experiences of the individual as well as their own personal values – they are largely independent of perceived quality of life and acceptance of the limb absence. Overall, the self-reported psychosocial health of individuals with limb absence is high regardless of prosthesis use or non-use (Biddiss and Chau 2008a). This supports the belief that individuals make the personal choice that maximizes their quality of life. As expected, prosthesis wearers report much higher levels of satisfaction with current prosthetic options than non-wearers. Should improvement in resources and prosthetic options be available, 75% of non-wearers would re-evaluate their decision not to adopt prosthesis use (Biddiss et al. 2007). Ultimately, the goal of an individual is constant: given the available resources, how can my needs best be met?

2.3 Prosthetic Technology: Need-Directed Design

For many individuals, a prosthesis is regarded in much the same light as a piece of clothing and this is a very apt analogy to envisage when considering its design. Imagine spending a day walking around in an uncomfortable pair of shoes; the embarrassment that might result should your clothes not perform as expected or fail during a critical moment; the frustration that you might feel if you were expected to choose one outfit to fit every occasion or did not have access to a change of clothes when doing the laundry. Prosthesis design exacts an extremely high standard of excellence to balance demands for comfort, function, durability, and affordability. The human hand, with its 20 degrees of freedom and over 17,000 sensors (Seow 1988), is by no means an easy act to follow and remains beyond the reach of current, albeit progressing, technology. Design tradeoffs are unavoidable and should be guided by consumer needs and priorities.

2.3.1 Consumer Design Priorities

Table 2.2 presents a list of focus areas for future design efforts compiled from feedback provided by consumers when asked to list their top five design priorities (Biddiss et al. 2007).

2.3.1.1 Design for Comfort

Consumers desire prostheses created for comfort. Regardless of device type, decreased weight is the number one priority on consumers' wish lists. The supporting structure

Table 2.2 Consumer design priorities for passive, body-powered, and electric prostheses

Priority ranking	Body-powered(N=47)	Passive(N=34)	Electric(N=77)	Overall(N=158)
1	Weight	Weight	Weight	Weight
2	Harness	Lifelike	Cost, Glove durability	Cost
3	Cost	Fit	Heat	Heat
4	Grip Strength	Fine motor	Sensory feedback	Lifelike
5	Sensory feedback	Heat	Lifelike	Sensory feedback
6	Fit	Cost	Fine motor skills	Harness
7	Heat	Colour match	Wrist function	Fit
8	Lifelike	Appearance under clothing	Frequency of unplanned movements	Fine motor skills
9	Reliability	Control of opening/ closing	Fit	Glove durability
10	Wrist function	Harness	Size	Wrist function

and weight distribution of current prosthetics differs greatly from that of the natural limb. As such, a prosthesis which is comparable in weight to the natural limb may still be perceived as unreasonably heavy for an individual with limb absence. Development of novel, light-weight materials, mini-actuator or "artificial muscles" (Del Cura et al. 2003), and batteries may lighten the prostheses of the future. For willing individuals, more invasive attachment strategies such as osseointegration may also provide more natural and integrated weight distribution (Branemark et al. 2001).

Uncomfortable temperatures and excess perspiration is another source of user dissatisfaction that is reported widely with all types of devices. Implantable electrodes (Troyk et al. 2007) in addition to those based on mechanomyography (Silva et al. 2005) may enable the use of softer, less restrictive sleeves and sockets with improved heat dissipation characteristics. Developments in surface electrodes, including textile-based sensors (Hoffmann and Ruff 2007) and ultra-sensitive electrodes that can detect through clothing (Matthews et al. 2007), may also facilitate greater prosthesis comfort. Wearers of body-powered prosthetics are also particularly concerned with harness discomfort, which is associated with medical complications such as blisters and upper body pain. Implantable myoelectric sensors may also provide more universally accessible muscle sites for prosthesis control, and present alternatives for individuals who are currently dissatisfied with the comfort of body-powered harnesses. Custom silicone sockets and improved fabrication techniques may also lead to a more comfortable and satisfactory fit (Uellendahl et al. 2006).

2.3.1.2 Design for Cost

The cost of prostheses and maintenance is another important grievance, especially in the design of active devices. Decreased costs would not only make these resources available to a greater number of individuals, they would also enable the purchase of back-up components and activity-specific devices that could enhance consumer satisfaction and quality of life. Several studies have suggested the benefits of providing multiple prostheses and greater opportunities for individuals with limb differences to participate in sports and recreational activities (Webster et al. 2001). Development of prosthetic devices composed of highly modular components (Gow et al. 2001; Kyberd et al. 2007) is one design approach that may help to address cost efficiency. Another is the growing availability of 3D surface digitizing technology and rapid prototyping which could reduce labour and time costs associated with customized fitting (Wong 2006). Low cost prosthetic options are also greatly needed in developing nations where prosthesis use and acceptance is largely inhibited by lack of appropriate medical and prosthetic equipment, inexperienced personnel and information provision, unsuitable amputation practices, monetary limitations, geographic barriers, and absence of government support (Bigelow et al. 2004). Efforts to meet this demand are ongoing (Sitek et al. 2004) and include initiatives such as the The Open Prosthetics Project (2008).

2.3.1.3 Design for Anthropomorphism

Consumers desire more life-like appearance and finger dexterity. Although the former is largely addressed by highly cosmetic silicone gloves, this technology is beyond the economic reach of many individuals, particularly those who need a durable, functional device for activities of daily life. A demand for more affordable, colour-fast, tear resistant, life-like cosmetic gloves is clearly evident. Efforts to address the desire for more natural movement and dexterity are focused on the development of multi-articulated prostheses (Fite, et al. 2008; Kyberd et al. 2001; Yang et al. 2004; Zollo et al. 2007), "artificial muscles" based on shape memory alloys (De Laurentis and Mavroidis 2002; dos Santos et al. 2003; Price et al. 2006), electroactive polymers (Biddiss and Chau 2008b) or mini-pneumatic/hydraulic actuators (Caldwell and Tsagarakis 2002; Kargov et al. 2008; Price et al. 2006), multi-functional control strategies that enable a variety of grasp types (Chan and Englehart 2003), and targeted reinnervation (wherein the residual nerves are redirected to the pectoral muscle which is used as a relay station to convey motor commands from the brain and to receive sensory information from the prosthetic hand) to enable simultaneous, thought-initiated, natural control and sensory feedback (Kuiken et al. 2004). The need for greater wrist function and control is also noted and is the focus of design efforts (Mustafa et al. 2006).

2.3.1.4 Design for Sensation

Sensory feedback is a final design priority of interest, particularly for consumers of active devices. Sensory mechanisms are valuable in determining the level of grasp required to manipulate objects, to reduce the cognitive load and need for visual attention, to prevent objects from slipping from one's grasp and improve reflex response, and to gather valuable tactile information. In addition to efforts to develop appropriate sensors to collect tactile and proprioceptive information from upper limb prosthetics (Biddiss and Chau 2006; Carpaneto et al. 2003; Cranny et al. 2005; Riso 1999; Zecca et al. 2004), targeted reinnervation has been demonstrated as one possible mechanism to provide a natural interface for sensory feedback (Kuiken et al. 2004). Although not appropriate for all individuals, this approach may be of particular interest to high level, traumatic amputees, for whom current prosthetic options are sub-par.

2.3.2 *Design for Function*

More and more, rehabilitation strategies are aimed at achieving functional goals (e.g. play hockey, prepare dinner independently) rather than physical metrics (e.g. range of motion, grip strength), as evident in recent outcome measures (Wright et al. 2003). It is therefore important to be aware of the activities that individuals with upper limb absence currently find challenging in their everyday lives. This knowledge can be used in the development of prosthetics and training strategies to alleviate frustrations and improve participation and independence. Table 2.3 presents a list of activities reported by individuals when asked to describe the challenges they face (Biddiss et al. 2007). Adult individuals with acquired limb absence, and those with limb absence at a higher level, reported a greater number of challenges. Almost all individuals who reported a large number of challenges made use of a prosthesis to aid in their daily life. Users and non-users were equally represented in the group of individuals who reported the absence of encountered challenges.

2.4 Enabling Resources: Meeting Needs

2.4.1 *Healthcare Services*

Satisfaction with healthcare and information services is, not surprisingly, lower amongst prosthesis non-wearers as compared to wearers.

Clinically, two strategies are extremely important for encouraging prosthesis acceptance and prolonged use:

1. *Timely fitting*. It has been established that individuals who are fitted with a prosthesis within 2 years of birth or within 6 months of amputation are significantly more likely to continue prosthesis use than those who are not (Biddiss and Chau 2008a). It is likely that individuals learn to adapt without a prosthesis when they are without one for an extended period of time, particularly at a young age. Frustration with an inconvenient and time ineffective system for prosthesis

Table 2.3 Challenging activities as reported by individuals with upper limb absence. (Reprinted with permission from Taylor & Francis (http://www.tandf.co.uk/journals), Biddiss et al. 2007)

Activity	Detailed description	Percentage of respondents who reported challenges (%)
Household chores	Repairs and household maintenance (i.e. car repairs, shoveling snow, gardening, electrical work); general housework (i.e. vacuuming, dishes, cleaning); use of tools (i.e. hammer, power tools, shovels); heavy lifting; climbing (i.e. ladders)	40
Sports	Cycling; swinging sports (i.e. golf, baseball, tennis); monkey bars/climbing; swimming; exercising; rock climbing; boating (i.e. canoeing, kayaking); ball sports (i.e. basketball, volleyball)	30
Hobbies	Playing a musical instrument (i.e. guitar, piano); motorbike and airplane control; woodworking and crafts	22
Activities of daily living	Food preparation and eating (cutting food, peeling, slicing); dressing (i.e. zippers, buttons, laces, pantyhose, ties); hair styling; typing; washing/personal hygiene; childcare; driving	19
Social activities	Intimacy (i.e. sex, hugging); clapping; shaking hands; passing through airport security; dancing	8
Occupational activities	Operating heavy machinery and large vehicles (i.e. farming equipment, trucks); training to be a doctor, surgeon, chemist etc.; law enforcement	6
Overall	No challenges encountered	16
	Everything is challenging	10

procurement may also dissuade individuals from adopting the technology. Every effort should be made to minimize delays associated with prosthesis funding approvals and/or lack of available expertise, resources, and/or information.

2. *Involvement in prosthesis selection*. Including the individual in the choice of prosthesis also greatly enhances the possibility that it will be acceptable and used (Biddiss and Chau 2008a). This finding is irrespective of the type of device selected. In participating in the choice of prosthesis, an individual may feel greater ownership of and autonomy in the decision. They may be able to better guide the selection of a device that is conducive to their needs and lifestyle. As such, it is imperative that clinicians consult with the individual to determine their personal goals and needs before prescribing a device. Adherence to strict fitting policies and structures that do not consider the unique individuality of each client is likely to lead to great dissatisfaction both with the prescribed prosthesis and the healthcare services provided. Many individuals would appreciate the opportunity to try different devices before incurring the full cost. This again suggests a need for more modular and low-cost components.

In addition, there is a strong desire for up-to-date and consistent information flow, particularly on prosthetic and non-prosthetic options (Biddiss and Chau 2007a). Individuals require aid in the formation of realistic expectations for their prosthesis and guidance throughout the process. Greater direction and access to peer support networks is particularly important for new amputees, new parents, and youths. Access to prosthetists, general practitioners, occupational therapists, and surgeons experienced in upper limb absence are important as the needs of individuals with upper limb absence vary greatly from the more prevalent lower limb absence. Unavailability of information resources and expertise can be extremely frustrating and discouraging for individuals and their families. This is particularly problematic for individuals located in rural areas (Rogers 1998) and also in developing nations (Bigelow et al. 2004). Increased electronic communications and videoconferencing as used by remote consulting services such as Biodesigns Inc., may be advantageous and provide greater access to non-local expertise and guidance.

2.4.2 Social Support Mechanisms

A strong social support system is essential to promoting quality of life and fostering acceptance of the limb difference.

1. *Family and peer support.* Social and familial networks are extremely important for the development of a healthy self-image, acceptance, and quality of life (Tyc 1992; Varni and Setoguchi 1993; Varni et al. 1992). The decision to fit or not to fit a young child can be an agonizing one for parents. On the one hand, most parents want their child to feel comfortable in their own body with or without a prosthesis and do not want to convey the message that the child needs to wear a device to feel accepted and "normal." Neither do they want to restrict healthy activities of play or cause the child undue discomfort or frustration. On the other hand, early use of a prosthesis may improve long-term acceptance of the device and relieve some of the pressure incurred by the contralateral limb. The relative tradeoffs of use or non-use can be difficult to balance for all individuals with upper limb absence. A great demand exists for peer support during these stages of transition, acceptance, and self-actualization. This is particularly true for individuals with acquired limb absence who face a different set of challenges with regard to acceptance and adjustment than those with congenital limb absence. There is also a desire for increased education of the general public with respect to limb absence and amputation to mitigate negative social behaviours such as staring, teasing, and negative assumptions regarding the functional capabilities of a person with a limb difference.
2. *More accessible funding opportunities.* Although psychosocial health is not related to the extent of prosthesis use reported, it is strongly correlated to availability of and access to resources. Individuals who are forced to make choices

Table 2.4 Consumer specified recommendations for prosthesis funding structures

Challenge	Consumers' needs
Need for full coverage	"More coverage. Most insurances pays 80% but the other 20% is brutal" [495]
Coverage for back-up and secondary devices	"Insurance paid for initial pros., but the deductible is so high that i can't afford replacement or repairs, so i need to be really careful of this one." [602]"Recognize that one single prosthesis purchase is NOT a lifetime solution." [108]
	"funding for sports to get children out and involved." [159]
	"more understanding from insurance companies. realizing the ongoing required maintenance...and the associated cost. the importance of backup -spare parts- for a bilateral amputee." [95]
Coverage for modern technologies	"Standardize the provision of prostheses so we don't have to fight with the insurance company every time because an electric hand is "too high tech." [137]
Coverage for passive, "cosmetic" prostheses	"Coverage, it is NOT cosmetic, I can not tie shoelaces or prepare supper if I do not have one." [212]
More efficient review process	"I would like to see Interference / red tape removed so amputees can try to get on with life. eg; having to prove 2 years after the fact your arm is missing. Reduce the amount of doctors you have to see before you get the ok to receive anything to do with the prosthesis." [360]
	"I know that my parents had a great deal of trouble with our healthcare providers while I was growing up and I often had to wait months for repairs and refitting because insurance was slow to permit it. I would like to see healthcare providers quicker to allow for prosthetic needs and less reluctant to cover new technology and new patient needs." [618]

based on economic constraints report lower quality of life. Grievances with respect to insurance coverage and funding structures are common, particularly in the United States. Challenges encountered and consumer reflections are listed in Table 2.4. Of the participants in this survey, 50% considered availability or cost to play at least a minor role in the decision not to wear a prosthesis.

2.5 Concluding Remarks

Prosthesis acceptance and use is driven by need. The choice to adopt or reject a prosthesis is made in such a way as to optimize quality of life and depends largely on personal comfort and perceived functional gain. User-centred design is essential to the development of prostheses that better meet consumer needs, particularly for individuals with high level and/or bilateral limb absence. Consumer design priorities are largely directed towards improving comfort, most notably by reducing the weight of current devices. Interest in life-like function and appearance, together with enhanced sensory feedback, is also apparent. Reduced costs and more efficient funding for prostheses and healthcare services are essential and will provide individuals with greater freedom in the selection of their prostheses, facilitated access to repairs and maintenance, and the possibility of procuring multiple and activity-specific prostheses. This is expected to increase overall prosthesis acceptance and quality of life. Clinical strategies aimed at (a) providing timely fitting and (b) involving consumers actively in the selection of their prosthesis may also improve prosthesis acceptance rates and consumer satisfaction. Lastly, consumers desire more in-depth, frequent, and accurate information pertaining to their prosthetic and non-prosthetic options and greater access to peer support networks.

References

Biddiss E, Chau T (2006) Electroactive polymeric sensors in hand prostheses, Bending response of an ionic polymer metal composite. Med Eng Phys 28:568–578

Biddiss E, Chau T (2007a) Upper limb prosthetics: critical factors in device abandonment. Am Arch Phys Med Rehabil 86(12):977–987

Biddiss E, Chau T (2007b) The roles of predisposing characteristics, established need, and enabling resources on upper extremity prosthesis use and abandonment. Disabil Rehabil: Assist Technol 2(2):71–84

Biddiss E, Chau T (2007c) Upper extremity prosthesis use and abandonment: A survey of the last 25 years. Prosthet Orthot Int 31(3):236–257

Biddiss E, Chau T (2008a) Multivariate prediction of upper limb prosthesis acceptance or rejection. Disabil Rehabil: Assist Technol 3(4):181–192

Biddiss E, Chau T (2008b) Dielectric elastomers as actuators for upper limb prosthetics, challenges and opportunities. Med Eng Phys 30(4):403–418

Biddiss E, Beaton D, Chau T (2007) Consumer design priorities for upper limb prosthetics. Disabil Rehabil: Assist Technol 2(6):346–357

Bigelow J, Korth M, Jacobs J, Anger N, Riddle M, Gifford J (2004) A picture of amputees and the prosthetic situation in Haiti. Disabil Rehabil 26(4):246–252

Branemark R, Branemark PI, Rydevik B, Myers RR (2001) Osseointegration in skeletal reconstruction and rehabilitation: a review. J Rehabil Res Dev 38(2):175–181

Caldwell DG, Tsagarakis N (2002) Biomimetic actuators in prosthetic and rehabilitation applications. Technol Health Care 10(2):107–120

Carpaneto J, Micera S, Zaccone F, Vecchi F, Dario P (2003) A sensorized thumb for force closed-loop control of hand neuroprostheses. IEEE Trans Neural Syst Rehabil Eng 11:346–353

Chan ADC, Englehart KB (2003) Continuous classification of myoelectric signals for powered prostheses using gaussian mixture models. In: Proceedings of the 25th annual international conference of the IEEE engineering in medicine and biology society. doi: 10.1109/IEMBS.2003.1280510

Cranny A, Cotton DPJ, Chappell PH, Beeby SP, White NM (2005) Thick-film force and slip sensors for a prosthetic hand. Sens Actuators A 123:162–171

De Laurentis K, Mavroidis C (2002) Mechanical design of a shape memory alloy actuated prosthetic hand. Technol Health Care 10:91–106

Del Cura VO, Cunha FL, Aguiar ML, Cliquet A (2003) Study of the different types of actuators and mechanisms for upper limb prostheses. Artif Organs 27(6):506–516

dos Santos CML, da Cunha FL, Dynnikov VI (2003) The application of shape memory actuators in anthropomorphic upper limb prostheses. Artif Organs 27(5):473–477

Fite KB, Withrow TJ, Shen X, Wait KW, Mitchell JE, Goldfarb M (2008) A gas-actuated anthropomorphic prosthesis for transhumeral amputees. IEEE Trans Robot 24(1):159–169

Gow DJ, Douglas W, Geggie C, Monteith E, Stewart D (2001) The development of the Edinburgh modular arm system. Proc Inst Mech Eng 215(3):291–298

Hoffmann KP, Ruff R (2007) Flexible dry surface-electrodes for ECG long-term monitoring. In: 29th annual international conference of IEEE engineering in medicine and biology society. doi: 10.1109/IEMBS.2007.4353650

Kargov A, Werner T, Pylatiuk C, Schulz S (2008) Development of a miniaturized hydraulic actuation system for artificial hands. Sens Actuators A Phys 141(2):548–557

Kuiken TA, Dumanian GA, Lipschutz RD, Miller LA, Stubblefield KA (2004) The use of targeted muscle reinnervation for improved myoelectric prosthesis control in a bilateral shoulder disarticulation amputee. Prosthet Orthot Int 28(3):245–253

Kyberd PJ, Light C, Chappell PH, Nightingale JM, Whatley D, Evans M (2001) The design of anthropomorphic prosthetic hands: a study of the Southampton Hand. Robotica 19:593–600

Kyberd PJ, Poulton AS, Sandsjo L, Jonsson S, Jones B, Gow D (2007) The ToMPAW modular prosthesis: A platform for research in upper-limb prosthetics. JPO J Prosthet Orthot 19(1):15–21

Matthews R, McDonald NJ, Hervieux P, Turner PJ, Steindorf MA (2007) A wearable physiological sensor suite for unobtrusive monitoring of physiological and cognitive state. In: 29th annual international conference of IEEE engineering in medicine and biology society. doi: 10.1109/IEMBS.2007.4353532

Mustafa SK, Yang G, Yeo SH, Lin W, Pham CB (2006) Development of a bio-inspired wrist prosthesis. In: 2006 IEEE conference on robotics, automation and mechatronics. doi: 10.1109/RAMECH.2006.252716

Price A, Jnifene A, Naguib HE (2006) Biologically inspired anthropomorphic arm and dextrous robot hand actuated by smart-material-based artificial muscles. In: Proceedings of the SPIE – The international society for optical engineering. doi: 10.1117/12.660471

Riso RR (1999) Strategies for providing upper extremity amputees with tactile and hand position feedback-moving closer to the bionic arm. Technol Health Care 7:401–409

Rogers JL (1998) Serving amputee patients in rural settings. Caring 17(9):32–33

Seow K (1988) Physiology of touch, grip, and gait. In: Webster J (ed) Tactile sensors for robotics and medicine. Wiley, New York

Silva J, Heim W, Chau T (2005) A self-contained mechanomyography-driven externally powered prosthesis. Arch Phys Med Rehabil 86(10):2066–2070

Sitek AJ, Yamaguchi GT, Herring DE, Willems CJ, Boninger D, Boninger RM (2004) Development of an inexpensive upper-extremity prosthesis for use in developing countries. J Prosthet Orthot 16(3):94–102

The Open Prosthetics Project (2008) http://openprosthetics.org/. Accessed 10 Dec, 2008

Troyk PR, DeMichele GA, Kerns DA, Weir RF (2007) IMES: an implantable myoelectric sensor. In: Proceedings of the 29th annual international conference of the IEEE engineering in medicine and biology society. doi: 10.1109/IEMBS.2007.4352644

Tyc VL (1992) Psychosocial adaptation of children and adolescents with limb deficiencies, A review. Clin Psychol Rev 12:275–291

Uellendahl JE, Mandacina S, Ramdial S (2006) Custom silicone sockets for myoelectric prostheses. J Prosthet Orthot 18(2):35–40

Varni JW, Setoguchi Y (1993) Effects of parental adjustment on the adaptation of children with congenital or acquired limb deficiencies. J Dev Behav Pediatr 14(1):13–20

Varni JW, Setoguchi Y, Rappaport LR, Talbot D (1992) Psychological adjustment and perceived social support in children with congenital/acquired limb deficiencies. J Behav Med 15(1):31–44

Webster JB, Levy CE, Bryant PR, Prusakowski PE (2001) Sports and recreation for persons with limb deficiency. Arch Phys Med Rehabil 82(3):S38–S44

Wong K (2006) Restoring lives with rapid prototyping. Cadalyst 23(7):16–18

Wright FV, Hubbard S, Naumann S, Jutai J (2003) Evaluation of the validity of the prosthetic upper extremity functional index for children. Arch Phys Med Rehabil 84(4):518–527

Yang J, Pena Pitarch E, Abdel-Malek K, Patrick A, Lindkvist L (2004) A multi-fingered hand prosthesis. Mech Mach Theory 39:555–581

Zecca M, Cappiello G, Sebastiani F, Roccella S, Vecchi F, Carrozza MC et al (2004) Experimental analysis of the proprioceptive and exteroceptive sensors of an underactuated prosthetic hand. Lect Notes Control Inf Sci 306:233–242

Zollo L, Roccella S, Guglielmelli E, Carrozza MC, Dario P (2007) Biomechatronic design and control of an anthropomorphic artificial hand for prosthetic and robotic applications. IEEE/ASME Trans Mechatron 12(4):418–429

Chapter 3
Ethical and Medico-Legal Issues in Amputee Prosthetic Rehabilitation

Jai Kulkarni

Abstract This chapter focuses on ethical and medico-legal issues in amputee prosthetic rehabilitation. Ethics is a critical evaluation of assumptions and arguments and is the study of what we "ought" to do. One ethical cluster of principles includes respect for autonomy, non malefience, beneficence and justice. Health care professionals "think" that they always do what is right for the patient, however in amputee rehabilitation and prosthetics with contracts with private companies there can be business pressures and resultant conflicts.

The primary duty of the clinician is to act in the best interests of the patient. Clinicians make better ethical decisions if they have a chance to think about them. It is only recently that we have begun to address ethical issues in amputee rehabilitation, with such attention previously focusing on acute care issues. Ethical dilemmas relate to goal setting, patient selection, resource allocation, teamwork issues and expectations of patients. There is an element of rationing in health service owing to a lack of resources and doctors are pushed into the role of gatekeepers. This chapter discusses a range of such issues as implicated in amputee prosthetic rehabilitation.

3.1 Introduction

Amputation or limb loss, whether in upper limb or lower limb is one of the most obvious manifestations of physical loss and physical disability, along with disruption of body image.

Amputation results from two main causative factors, namely a congenital deficiency or an acquired causation. A congenital limb deficiency is one that is present in a child born with either deficiency of the upper limb or the lower limb or a multiple limb affection.

J. Kulkarni
Department of Rehabilitation Medicine, DSC, University Hospitals of South Manchester, M20 1LB, UK
e-mail: jai.kulkarni@uhsm.nhs.uk

C. Murray (ed.), *Amputation, Prosthesis Use, and Phantom Limb Pain: An Interdisciplinary Perspective*, DOI 10.1007/978-0-387-87462-3_3,

The causation of lower limb amputations in the United Kingdom has changed in the last 70 years, from trauma subsequent to the Second World War to dysvascularity as the main factor. Dysvascularity related to peripheral vascular disease and diabetes is now noted to be the most common cause of lower limb amputations in the UK.

Data from the 2005 to 2006 National Amputee Statistical Database Group (NASDAB) in the United Kingdom indicates that dysvascularity is the cause of lower limb amputation in 75% of presentations. By rough estimates there are approximately 50,000 lower limb amputees in the United Kingdom and recent NASDAB data indicates that 5,000 amputees were referred to various Disablement Services Centres for amputee/prosthetic rehabilitation in 2005/2006. Of these, 50% were over the age of 65 years of age and 25% were over 75 years of age. The median age for males was noted to be 65 years, for females 69 years. Lower limb amputations accounted for 91% of referrals, with 5% being for upper limb amputations, and 4% in the congenital/other causative factors group (NASDAB 2005).

In lower limb amputees, the causation is mainly dysvascularity whereas it is mainly trauma related in upper limb amputees. The lower limb amputees do have significant associated co-morbidities of impairment of their cardiac, cerebral, respiratory and musculo skeletal system. They suffer a "double whammy" with the compounded factor of overall decrease in survival rates as compared to the normal cohort. In the United Kingdom, following limb amputation, patients undergo a process of rehabilitation including prosthetic rehabilitation which involves multidisciplinary assessment, fitting, maintenance and repairs of the prostheses.

The process of amputee rehabilitation goes through the following phases:

(a) Pre-amputation phase.
(b) Amputation surgery phase.
(c) Post-amputation phase.
(d) Prosthetic rehabilitation phase.
(e) Maintenance rehabilitation phase.

These are the phases for the acquired amputee, whereas in the patient with congenital factors the phases are mainly of prosthetic rehabilitation and maintenance – phases d and e. The length of amputation phase depends on the nature of the causation. In trauma related amputation, this is a sudden event, whereas in the elderly cohort with PVD/dysvascularity with or without diabetes this could be a long drawn out phase. The amputation surgery phase is a specialised area of work which is outside the discussion of this chapter apart from the fact that there are ethical issues relating to the consent for amputation which will be covered in the latter section.

The post amputation phase is usually a period of convalescence or recovery followed by the prosthetic rehabilitation phase, which currently involves referral to the Disablement Services Centre team.

The maintenance rehabilitation phase is also important as, unlike for many other health problems, the episode of care does not finish, as in elective surgery procedures similar to routine hernia repair. Subsequent to hernia repair the episode of care finishes and on balance the patient hardly ever sees the surgeon subsequent to hospital discharge. In the case of an amputee or a child with congenital limb deficiency, the person needs lifelong follow up and hence there are issues pertaining to establishing a relationship with the clinical team to assist with ongoing rehabilitation.

As with any other clinical area, amputee rehabilitation medicine involves numerous clinical issues of autonomy – for example, consent, beneficence, non-malefience, accountability for reasonableness by the clinical team, the patient–clinician relationship and distributive costs and other related ethical and medico-legal issues. It would be inappropriate to consider all these issues in detail, as although they raise interesting ethical areas of discussion, these are no different from any other area of medicine and are not peculiar to limb loss. However it would be appropriate to cover specific areas as these issues can be part of the unique situation pertaining to the amputee.

Healthcare professionals "think" that they "always do what is right for the patient". The primary duty of the clinician is to always act in the best interests of the patient. The conflicts between the needs of the individuals, the best interests of the family and the expectations of society need to be addressed. As professionals we are charged with putting the patient first but with lack of true research and biased marketing, which one of us can make the right call? Overall, almost all people, including health professional, make better ethical decisions if they have a chance to think about them. Specifically doctors and other healthcare professionals should be able to justify the value judgementsand also the scientific judgements that they make. In the UK, it is only recently that we have begun to address ethical issues in Amputee Rehabilitation Medicine, with such attention previously focusing almost exclusively on Acute Medicine. In the remainder of this chapter a range of such issues, as they arise in amputee prosthetic rehabilitation, will be discussed.

3.2 Attitudes Pertaining to Autonomy: Consent

The word autonomy is derived from the Greek words autos meaning self and nomy meaning rule. Autonomy is the capacity to direct and control one's own life. English law endorses the patient's right to autonomy and recognises the value of informed consent (Bauchamp and Childress 1994).

Respect for the patient requires a patient's autonomous consent to be obtained before any treatment or procedure involving the patient can be carried out, and no consent will be autonomous unless it is a fully informed consent. Hence any healthcare professional who fails to make a full and frank disclosure of all the facts or prognosis about a patient's condition, before obligatory consent to proceed, would not have valid consent. Any attempt to treat a patient without valid consent would be treating the patient with scant respect and would violate his or her autonomy (Harris 1997).

A possible example is that of a patient in the pre-amputation phase when admitted in a toxic state, especially in an elderly patient with severe circulatory problems compounded by infection and a liable lower limb. In such a case limb salvage with reconstructive surgery is not an option but getting a truly informed consent from the patient who is in a toxic state is a difficult proposition. The treating team then needs to involve the next of kin and, within reason, try and explain to them the need for an amputation as a life saving measure. Consent can then be obtained from next of kin. In an emergency situation, the treating consultant needs to liaise with a colleague consultant so that the two consultants can decide and come to a consensus that intervention is needed on a clinical needs basis and best interest basis for a life threatening situation, and the team can proceed with necessary amputation surgery on a "best interest" principle.

Another difficult area is when an adult patient (over the age of 18 years) with a life threatening lower limb condition chooses not to consent for the amputation. If this patient is deemed to be mentally competent and shown to have functional capacity, then it is accepted that he or she would be able to refuse treatment albeit it would lead to worsening of his or her clinical condition. Overall the patient's wishes have to be respected.

It is a well-established rule of common law that for public interest reasons, reasonable or proper medical treatment stands completely outside criminal law. In common law there is a presumption of capacity and this can be rebuffed only if, on the functional assessment, the patient is unable to make his or her own decision (Mental Capacity 2005).

In the situation where a teenager, namely a teenager between the ages of 15–17, disagrees with his or her parents regards to treatment, then in such a case the Gillick Principle needs to be applied. This refers to a ruling by the House of Lords in the UK that children under the age of 16 who fully understand what is proposed, along with its implications, are competent to give consent to medical treatment. If the teenager is Gillick competent, he or she can decide either to undergo the operative treatment or take the decision till at a later stage. The decision to follow this approach must be taken on clinical grounds and depends heavily on the severity and the permanence of the proposed treatment plan. On the other hand, the teenager though not obviously an adult of consenting age can give consent to the clinical team even though he or she is under the age of 16 if heor she is deemed to be Gillick competent (Gillick V West Norfolk and Wisbech Area Health Authority 1986).

The guiding principle is that the actual needs of the patient should drive the doctor–patient relationship, recognising that over time these needs may change. It is often noted that the needs the patient starts off with are not necessarily those he or she ends up with. This is particularly true in the elderly cohort of patients as there is an element of prejudice to age, albeit tacit at times, in the health service. To some extent limitations are put on patients in the elderly age spectrum are neglected and preference is given to the younger patient. Overall an equitable practice is to be encouraged in such situations, and the approach, has to be need-based rather than age-based in their entirety.

3.3 Non-malefience

Pertaining to amputee rehabilitation, a holistic approach by the multidisciplinary team would avoid potential problems. At a clinical level in the case of a child with congenital limb deficiency, parents and extended family can exert undue pressure on the clinician to introduce heavy electronic prosthesis at an early stage, albeit with a penalty of extra weight on the residual limb/stump. From a clinical point of view the heavy prosthesis could cause disruption to the growing bone and further compound the deformity in the child whilst trying to fit in with the parents' wishes.

3.4 Justice: Resource Allocation and Distributive Costs

Doctors are often forced to play the role of a gate keeper by proxy. Though they are placed in an awkward situation, they must try and do their best for the individual patient (beneficence) whilst also controlling budgets and assuring maximal clinical activity. Resource allocation decisions in healthcare are rife with moral disagreements and a transparent deliberate process is necessary to establish the legitimacy and fairness of such decisions (Daniels 2000).

Clinical priority related decision rest on two types of information, the severity of the patient's condition (prognosis without intervention) and the expected outcome (prognosis with intervention). Clinicians can help support priority setting by stopping procedures that have little evidence of effectiveness. Priority setting is an integral part of daily practice in many clinical specialties. Non-clinical considerations are also important, namely characteristics of area of residence, religion, ethnicity and social status.

The ability to pay should be considered irrelevant, though recently the health Minister via the Department of Health has been addressing the issue of top up payments, especially in cancer care. Age may become relevant if clinicians must choose life extending procedures.

There is a tacit but nonetheless definitive element of rationing pertaining to the area of amputee prosthetic rehabilitation and long term follow up. Rationing at times is explicit but also has a notable implicit element. Rationing can occur at four levels, namely, at the level of the Government–Department of Health, at the level of the Health Authority–Strategic Authorities, at service level and at the individual clinician level. Overall although there is tacit rationing, clinical priority settings should be the platform from which a reasoned approach of management is essential. On the other hand the question is always of resources and linked to this is the lack of resources but the presence of clinical need. In this situation clinical priority setting and setting up of guidelines on the issue of prosthetic componentry is beneficial.

Non-selected patients need to be informed of the availability of any follow up evaluation to determine further review or selection. The ethical dilemma of patient selection in the post-amputation phase is between in-patient amputee care and out-patient amputee care. On a clinical prioritising basis this should be on medical factors mainly relating to prognostic issues. But unfortunately non-medical factors come into play namely post code approach, age related approach, and unfortunate resource issue of bed availability. We should endeavour to maintain a position of equipoise.

Another ethical dilemma is the issue of goal setting both by the patient and by the clinical team. Goals are the functional outcomes that the patient and the team strive to achieve. This obviously involves the patient, the rehabilitation team, the family and society as well, as we all value independence and self sufficiency. A high premium is placed on physical mobility and cosmesis of the prosthesis. There can be ethical dilemmas between various members of the multidisciplinary and the interdisciplinary team. There can be conflict issues within the team or between the team and the patient because of unrealistic patient expectations. One way forward would be to do a group think of these issues involving all concerned. Steps to bring about a concert of moral interest within a team would be to address common moral issues, rational discussion and value clarification to develop a moral decision making method. Acceptable moral policies need to be drawn from common experiences.

With regard to the issue of accountability for reasonableness, it is appropriate to address the areas of relevance, evidence based and resource led, with a view to also addressing the constraints that exist. Publicity of new technologies that are being introduced, on a regular basis in prosthetic technology, needs to be addressed.

3.5 Rationing

In prosthetic rehabilitation there is some rationing as a result of the high cost and scarcity of certain items in particular, pertaining to the high cost technological prosthetic items, for example a myo-electric prosthesis for upper limb amputees and customised computerised knee units for lower limb amputees. There is growing concern regarding the high costs of high definition silicone cosmeses, the material which covers the endoskeletal part of the artificial limb to give a lifelike appearance.

Non-acute specialities like rehabilitation medicine, along with other areas of medicine like pain medicine, palliative care medicine and community care medicine, fall behind the acute specialties such as cardiology, paediatrics and cancer medicine as developmental monies are more likely to be allocated to these acute areas.

It would be appropriate to consider the concept of fairness to determine how societies' resources are distributed equitably. The philosopher John Rawls' notion of fairness to determine what is just evokes the concept that he calls the equally poised position, in which people choose the principles of a just society from a position where no one knows his or her place in society, social status or ability to pay. With this veil of ignorance, resources can be distributed equally, unless any unequal distribution of any or all is to everyone's advantage, and argues that society is better off only when it makes least well off people better off.

3.6 Best Interest Principle: High-Tech or Low-Tech

Patients irrespective of age and health seem drawn to the promises of high-tech prosthetic technology even though the technology may be overkill, as they see this as a psychological boost. They often make comments such as "give me the best system, even if I don't need all of its features". As noted earlier, there is tacit but nonetheless definitive rationing of resources in the health service. It would be inappropriate ethically and morally to distribute high-tech resources like extremely expensive components to a small group of amputees whilst denying reasonable technologically available prescriptions for a larger number of amputees. On the other hand, it would be ethically and morally wrong to deny a young, fit working age amputee the ability to realize his or her potential in work, vocation and sports potential if they were to use one system for work and an advanced technological sports system to improve their sporting prowess.

With the introduction of computerised knee units, which do increase the element of safety and improve the gait pattern and lead to decreased energy expenditure, there has been a clamour for these units from patients with limited ambulation potential. Unfortunately the private prosthetic industry tends to glamorise these components and because of high costs it is difficult to have access to them on a regular basis via the limited budget of the National Health Service-led clinical set-ups in the UK. One such example is the introduction of computerised C-Leg units for above knee amputees, and another is the concept of introducing Proprio feet for the lower limb amputees. In my opinion it is more appropriate for the approach to be clinically-led and evidence-based medicine-led. Unfortunately there can be judicial interference with professional judgement and allocation of resources. On the other hand in a judicial review of statutory services providing equipment was a case that was deliberated by Lord Denning of the Court of Appeals in 1980, where the judgement passed was that the NHS could not be expected to deliver every last piece of high technology item or state of art treatment.

Against this backdrop there is an increasing litigation and culture of blame in our society. The law has become increasingly intrusive in health care service delivery areas. Although there are only a finite number of medico-legal cases in amputee proshetic rehabilitation compared to acute medicine areas, there is nonetheless an increasing concern in this area. If there is definitive negligence which is proven by harm occurring to a patient because of breach of duty and lack of care, then it would be most appropriate for that patient to be compensated for this harm that he or she has suffered because of improper, or substandard clinical management. In obvious cases the assumption of negligence is clear with evidential burden – res ipsa loquitus –things speak for themselves. The Medical Devices Regulation Authority, recently changed to the Medical and Health Regulatory Authority, has indicated that artificial limbs are Medical Devices. If there is any material contribution to an accident resulting from a faulty artificial limb then the issue of product liability and the Consumer Act 1987 can come into play. There is strict liability for defective products. Such items in prosthetic technology are CE marked but unfortunately a

CE mark is not a cast iron guarantee of safety. It is a mark of harmonised standards within the European Community/Conformity European. Breach of duty in relation to equipment can lead to criminal liability or civil liability.

In the case of faulty mechanisms in the artificial limb prosthesis, for example, if there is a faulty semi-automatic knee lock and the patient falls sustaining bony injury, and it can be proven that the faulty mechanism caused the fall, then the patient can seek legal redress. On the other hand, if the patient tampered or interfered with the knee lock mechanism, and in effect it can be proven that the setting at the time of delivery of the artificial limb was appropriate and that the method was demonstrated to the patient, and if there is clear evidence of tampering, then there is no question of legal redress.

If a non-compliant patient self-adjusts the setting of the foot and ankle of the prosthetic set-up and then sustains a related injury and if the records/clinical records are up to date then there is no case for legal redress. There needs to be reasonable documentation in the case notes and details that standard protocols were followed up.

The area of artificial limb prostheses and the delivery of these are somewhat unique in the NHS in that prosthetic companies are sub-contracted to the NHS via a particular Trust. Hence, on one hand the entire clinical team is an NHS Trust Team whereas the prosthetic team is employed by a private company which is sub-contracted to the NHS. In most large centres these are well integrated teams but in some smaller centres there is an obvious separation and divide between "them and us". With concerted effort, prosthetists have now integrated into the Healthcare Professional Council. Patients cannot successfully sue healthcare professionals simply because they experience a bad outcome, as most adverse outcomes in this area result from a normal sequelae of progressive pathology. To some extent problems can occur because of non-negligent errors in professional judgement.

For patients to succeed in healthcare mal-practice litigation they must prove that a legitimate basis exists pertaining to professional negligence, standard of care issues, duty of care issues, intentional misconduct, breach of contract and/or product liability. Mal-practice can also relate, and does so in the majority of cases, to professional negligence or substandard care. In rare cases malpractice claims can result from premises related liability namely vicarious liability issues because of unsafe environment. Overall malpractice issues in the prosthetics and orthotics industry are still very rare. In my opinion, establishing a clinical liability risk management group to look at the likely issues before or as they happen would lead to resolution in most if not all such cases.

3.7 Withdrawal of Prostheses

Withdrawal of prostheses from the patient is justified if there are concerns regards cognitive impairment and safety. Temporary withdrawal of prostheses can be initiated in cases of clinical necessity, relating to either stump healing issues or temporary impairment or incapacity during a notable illness episode.

Lastly, good clinical practice requires that value judgements are properly analysed and assessed just as scientific and technical evidence should be properly evaluated and decisions should be evidence-based.

3.8 Concluding Comments

In this chapter a range of ethical and medico–legal issues arising in amputee prosthetic rehabilitation have been presented and discussed. Although these issues have been discussed here many in relation to the context of service provision in the United Kingdom, these issues have broad applicability to other countries and contexts of service delivery. It is therefore hoped that this chapter serves to stimulate further discussion among clinical and health professionals involved in amputee prosthetic rehabilitation.

References

Bauchamp PC, Childress JE (1994) Principles of biomedical ethics, 4th edn. Oxford University Press, Oxford, pp 190–192
Daniels N (2000) Accountability for reasonableness. Br Med J 321:1300
Gillick V (1986) West Norfolk and Wisbech Area Health Authority and another 3 All ER 402 (HL)
Harris J (1997) A value of life: an introduction to medical ethics. Routledge, Great Britain, pp 205–206
Mental Capacity Act (2005) Crown copyright. London
NASDAB (2005) National amputee statistical database, crown copyright, Edinburgh. Accessed from website http://www.nasdab.co.uk

Chapter 4
Monitoring of Upper Limb Prosthesis Activity in Trans-Radial Amputees

Mohammad Sobuh, Laurence Kenney, Phil Tresadern, Martin Twiste, and Sibylle Thies

Abstract There has been a shift in rehabilitation medicine from conventional evaluation procedures towards more quantitative approaches. However, up to now, a quantitative evaluation procedure for upper limb prostheses that is applicable outside of the laboratory or clinical environment has not been established. The requirement for such a procedure arises from the findings of a number of recent studies suggesting that unilateral trans-radial amputees do not involve their prosthesis in task performance in real life situations, even if they are able to demonstrate the use of the prosthesis in the clinical environment. This suggests that laboratory, or clinic-based assessments are limited in the information they provide to clinicians or designers of new prostheses. Further, self-report approaches, such as questionnaires or interviews rely on accurate recall and reporting by subjects, an approach that has been shown to be flawed in other rehabilitation and public health domains.

Therefore, this chapter reports a study investigating the feasibility of quantifying the nature and duration of tasks performed with a myoelectric prosthesis by means of an activity monitor. It was hypothesised that by monitoring the prosthesis hand opening and closing it may be possible to identify the manipulation phase. Such information could be used to segment acceleration signals, measured from arm-located accelerometers, which may contain information characterising the task(s) being performed and differentiate it/them from other tasks. The results of this study indicate that, by using a neural network classifier, customised for each user, acceleration signals measured during the manipulation phase of task performance could accurately characterise the task being performed. The implications of these findings and future work are discussed here.

L. Kenney
Centre for Rehabilitation and Human Performance Research, Brian Blatchford building, University of Salford, Salford M6 6PU, UK
e-mail: l.p.j.kenney@salford.ac.uk

C. Murray (ed.), *Amputation, Prosthesis Use, and Phantom Limb Pain: An Interdisciplinary Perspective*, DOI 10.1007/978-0-387-87462-3_4,

4.1 Upper Limb Prostheses: Background

Every year in the UK approximately 200–300 upper limb amputees are referred to prosthesis fitting centres (NASDAB 2005) (Fig. 4.1). One of the most common types of upper limb amputation and the focus of the work presented in this chapter, is unilateral and trans-radial, in which hand and wrist function are completely lost and the ability to rotate the forearm is severely restricted. As the anatomical hand and wrist are key to the acquisition, manipulation and release of objects, as well as the proprioceptive inputs from the surrounding environment, their loss represents a major reduction in functional capability.

Three types of prosthesis are used in an attempt to restore the lost functions, namely, the body-powered prosthesis, cosmetic prosthesis, and myoelectric prosthesis. As its name suggests, the *body-powered prosthesis* (Fig. 4.2) is controlled by the motion of the proximal joints of the amputated side. The control system uses the

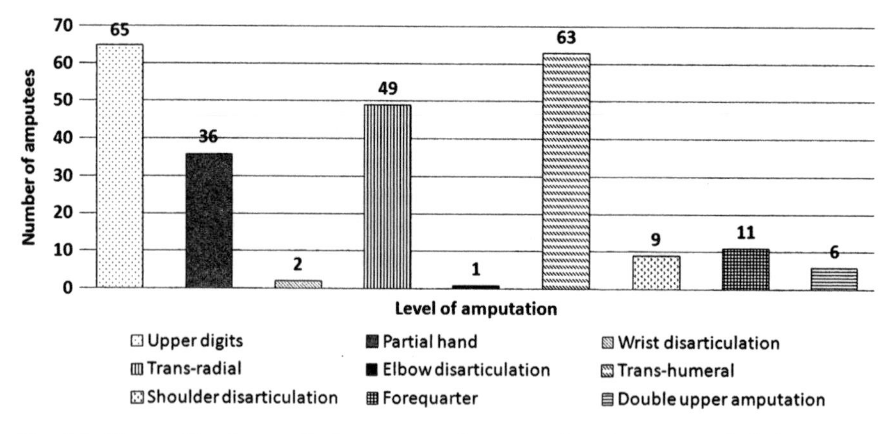

Fig. 4.1 The profile of upper limb amputees who were referred to prosthesis fitting centres in the UK in 2005/06. (Adapted from [NASDAB 2005])

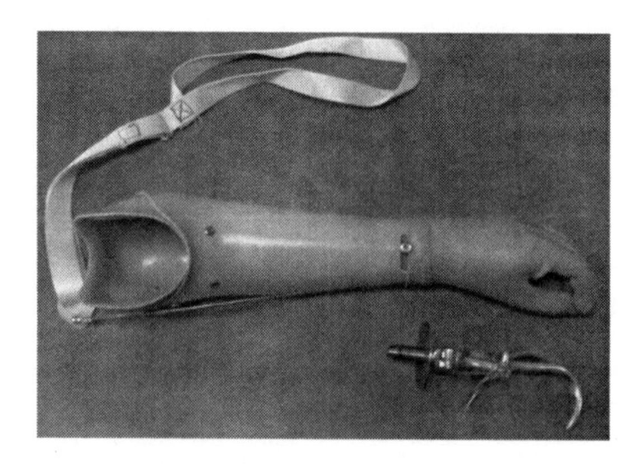

Fig. 4.2 A body-powered prosthesis, including harnessing straps and two different prehensors

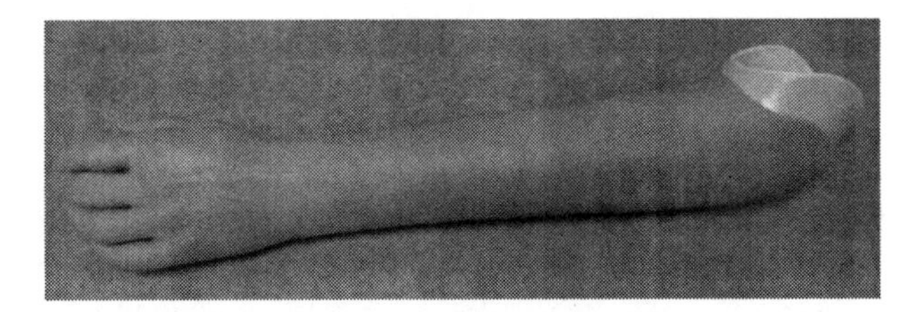

Fig. 4.3 A cosmetic prosthesis

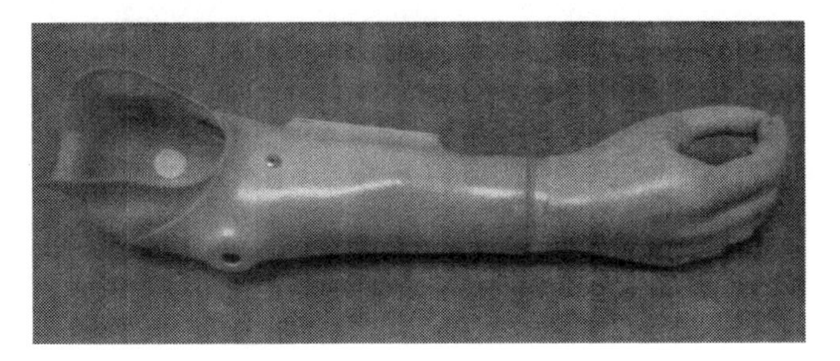

Fig. 4.4 A myoelectric prosthesis

motion of the harnessed shoulder(s) to pull a Bowden cable that, in case of a trans-radial prosthesis, operates a prehensor (the terminal device) (Smith et al. 2004).

When the cosmetic appearance, rather than the functionality, of the prosthesis is of primary importance to the amputee a *cosmetic prosthesis* (Fig. 4.3) is likely to be prescribed (Meier and Atkins 2004). Cosmetic prostheses are those designed to restore the appearance of the missing part(s) (i.e. shape, colour and texture), but usually provide no controllable moving parts (Meier and Atkins 2004).

The *myoelectric prosthesis* (Fig. 4.4) makes use of the electrical activity of contracting muscles (the electromyographic or EMG signals) at an appropriate site on the remaining musculature to control a battery-powered, motorised terminal device (a hand or a split hook) and/or wrist (Muzumdar 2004). Typically, the EMG signals, collected via socket-located electrodes, are amplified then rectified and filtered to provide a signal suitable for use with a threshold, or continuous control scheme.

4.2 Justification for the Study

The ultimate role of the prosthesis is to restore both lost function and cosmesis to a level that is available to a non-amputee so that he/she can achieve the normal, wide range of upper limb activities of daily living with minimal effort (Meier and Atkins 2004). This, however, is not fully possible with the current prostheses (Meier and Atkins 2004).

Although it can be argued that the limited functionality available with the current prostheses is probably a significant improvement over what was available in previous decades, the literature suggests that the technology remains far from ideal. In particular, recent publications suggest that amputees generally perform unilateral tasks with their non-amputated limb (Fraser 1998; Hermansson et al. 2005; Light et al. 2002). Further, they not only tend to rely more on the non-amputated side when performing bimanual tasks but also tend to perform such tasks in a more repeatable manner than healthy controls (Black et al 2005; Jones and Davidson 1999). All of these factors are believed to be consistent with an increased risk of cumulative trauma problems in the non-amputated side (Black et al 2005). These observations are supported by the high incidence of injuries related to overuse and associated pain in the non-amputated arm (Black et al 2005; Gambrell 2008; Jones and Davidson 1999). It is therefore reasonable to assume that, despite all improvements achieved in the upper limb prosthetic field over recent decades, upper limb prostheses, and arguably myoelectric prostheses in particular, are still used to only a limited extent by amputees in their daily lives.

As will be discussed in detail later in this chapter, upper limb prostheses are still largely evaluated using questionnaires and/or interviews, or laboratory-based tests. Such approaches may not accurately reflect either the range of tasks an amputee is able to accomplish with a prosthesis or how often an amputee uses the prosthesis in everyday situations. This limits the accuracy with which new upper limb prostheses or amputee training approaches can be evaluated. The study reported in this Chapter addresses this problem by investigating the potential for monitoring the activity type and frequency of use of upper limb prostheses in daily life. More specifically, the goal of the work was to demonstrate the feasibility of using signals from arm and/or prosthesis-located accelerometers, together with information on the opening of the prosthetic hand to identify the nature and duration of upper limb activities. The focus is initially on myoelectric prostheses but the approach is generalisable to other devices.

4.3 Upper Limb Prostheses and Their Evaluation

4.3.1 Introduction

Evaluation is the act of ascertaining the value or worth of an object. Clearly, the value of a prosthesis to its user is dependent not only on the technical features of the prosthesis, but also on psychological, societal and possibly other factors as well. Despite the complexity of prosthesis evaluation, it is nevertheless possible to develop tools that quantify certain aspects of the problem. As this study focuses on the functional aspects of the prosthetic hand, the value or worth of an upper limb prosthesis in functional terms can therefore be considered to be the extent to which it restores absent functionality, combined with the degree to which amputees make use of this additional function in their daily life.

Functionality can be defined as the ability to perform desired tasks or activities (Light et al 1999; 2002). In the context of upper limb prostheses, functionality is most often measured in terms of the ability to perform "Activities of Daily Living" (ADLs) that would normally involve the upper limb (Light et al. 2002), such as dressing, eating, toileting and hygiene (Weaver et al. 1988). *Usage* is reflected in the frequency/duration of prosthetic use and/or wearing patterns (Pruitt et al. 1996).

Functionality and usage are both central to the overall evaluation process (Burger et al. 2004; Wright et al. 1995). In the section below we report on the two approaches to prosthesis evaluation and highlight the inherent limitations of both, notably the absence of direct observation of prosthesis use and functionality during daily life. This is followed by a section introducing the topic of activity monitoring that has been used to gather such data in other applications. Finally, we propose a new approach; activity monitoring of upper limb prostheses.

4.3.2 Current Approaches to Prosthesis Evaluation

4.3.2.1 Questionnaires, Interviews and Clinical Records

The usage and/or functionality of upper limb prostheses in every-day life have traditionally been assessed from information obtained by postal questionnaires (Burger and Marincek 1994; Gaine et al 1997; Millstein et al. 1986; Wright et al. 1995; Roeschlein and Domholdt 1989), phone interviews (Thornby and Krebs 1992; Pezzin et al. 2004), or personal interviews (Kejlaa 1993; Northmore-Ball et al. 1980) and/or from reviewing patients' prosthetic records (Malone et al. 1984).

Usage has typically been estimated by asking the users to report either the frequency/duration of prosthesis usage (Kejlaa 1993; Silcox et al. 1993) or, the wearing pattern/length of time worn (Gaine et al. 1997; Malone et al 1984). Detailed definitions of the frequency/duration of "use" have included the period during which the terminal device was activated (Kejlaa 1993) and the period spent performing tasks, regardless of the status of the terminal device (van Lunteren et al. 1983). Both of these definitions have some merit but using a questionnaire, or interview as a measurement tool provides, at best, an approximation to the real data (Northmore-Ball et al. 1980). Further, such an approach is unlikely to yield detailed and reliable data on the type of activities carried out with a prosthesis. Estimating the wearing pattern alone is clearly of limited use for prosthesis evaluation, as it is insensitive to how the tasks are being performed.

Functionality is rarely clearly defined in the upper limb prosthetics literature. Previous researchers have chosen a variety of different terms that appear to relate to functionality in questionnaire/interview based studies. These include, for example, "the ability to perform activities" (Fraser 1998; Pruitt et al 1996; 1998; 1999) "the ease of performance with the prosthesis" (Wright et al 2003) and the "value of the prosthesis" (Northmore-Ball et al. 1980). Clearly, the answers to such questions, although of significant interest, are limited by their inherent subjectivity. Factors related to prosthetic use and wear have also been linked to functionality (Millstein et al. 1986; Pezzin et al. 2004; Roeschlein and Domholdt 1989; Weaver et al. 1988). Other descriptors include the number of ADLs that are normally performed with a prosthesis Light et al. 1999; Silcox et al. 1993; van Lunteren et al. 1983). However, as is the case with measures of prosthesis use/ usage, using self-report to estimate quantitative data on specific prosthesis ADL performance, or pre-amputation performance provides at best an indirect estimate.

4.3.2.2 Direct-Observation Based Functionality Tests

Certain detailed aspects of evaluation such as dexterity, manipulating ability and spontaneity ("the tendency to use the prosthesis without considerable intention from the user") (Light et al. 1999; http://www.unb.ca/biomed/unb_test-of-prosthetics-function.pdf 2008) cannot be properly addressed by self-report. Therefore, a number of direct observation studies have been conducted involving the use of standardised tests. Such studies are normally run either under structured (Light et al 2002; Thornby and Krebs 1992) or semi-structured (http://www.unb.ca/biomed/unb_test-of-prosthetics-function.pdf 2008; Bagley et al. 2006) conditions. Typically, they involve the performance of a set of upper limb tasks, which the experimenter/clinician scores on an ordinal or interval scale.

Many of the older studies used generic upper limb tests (Agnew 1981; Bergman et al. 1992; Edelstein and Berger 1993) but there also exist four tests specifically developed for prosthesis evaluation, namely: the UNB (http://www.unb.ca/biomed/unb_test-of-prosthetics-function.pdf 2008), SHAP (Light et al. 2002) ACMC (Hermansson et al. 2005; 2006) and UBET test (Bagley et al 2006). Direct-observation tests, such as those listed previously, can show how well an amputee functions with his/her prosthesis under laboratory conditions and hence can directly measure elements of functionality. However, the ability of individuals to make use of their prosthesis under controlled conditions provides no direct information on their performance with the prosthesis in daily life (Fraser 1998; van Lunteren et al. 1983).

4.3.2.3 Conclusion

To date, a measure that is able to comprehensively evaluate both the functionality of upper limb prostheses and the usage in a real-life setting is not known to the authors. Although the scope of the evaluation process could be broadened by using both a questionnaire in combination with an observational test (Buffart et al. 2006; Burger et al. 2004; Wright 2006) such an approach would be very time-consuming. More importantly, it would still be limited by the absence of direct observational data in a real life situation. As will be discussed in the following section, activity monitoring is a potential solution to this problem.

4.3.3 Activity Monitoring

4.3.3.1 Background

Activity Monitoring is the continuous observing and recording of activities in a free-living environment by means of an "Activity Monitor" which typically consists of one or more wearable sensors, a power source and a data logger or communication device (Vega-Gonzalez and Granat 2005). Over the past decades, many activity monitors have been developed and tested for validity and reliability (Culhane et al. 2005; Godfrey et al. 2008). Application areas include movement of both the lower (Busse et al. 2004; Coleman et al. 1999) and upper (Schasfoort et al. 2006; Uswatte et al. 2000, 2005; Vega-Gonzalez and Granat 2005) limbs, in healthy individuals and individuals with disabilities (Busse et al. 2004; Coleman et al. 1999; Hansson et al 2006; Schasfoort et al. 2006; Uswatte et al. 2000, 2005) including lower limb amputees (Bussmann et al. 1998). A number of these devices are now commercially available and are being intensively and successfully used in many applications, including the evaluation of public health and rehabilitation programmes (Godfrey et al. 2008).

4.3.3.2 Sensor Technologies

Over recent years, sensors for activity monitoring applications have become both significantly smaller and cheaper (Culhane et al. 2005). These sensors include microelectromechanical (MEMS) accelerometers and gyroscopes, electronic goniometers and pressure sensors (Vega-Gonzalez and Granat 2005). Of these, the accelerometer is probably the most widely used in activity monitoring (Godfrey et al. 2008). It consists of a mass suspended on a compliant element. Gravitational and inertial forces acting on the mass cause the compliant element to deflect and the output is derived from measurement of this deflection. Suitably processed output can be used to estimate the accelerometer's linear acceleration, inclination (when stationary) and/or its magnitude and frequency of vibration. Accelerometers vary in measurement transduction technology, size, measuring sensitivity and number of axes. Typical accelerometers for human motion monitoring are now mm-scale devices that cost only a few pounds and require no more than μA to operate (e.g. http://www.analog.com).

4.3.3.3 Lower Limb and Whole Body Activity Monitors

Many physical impairments adversely affect both the ability to perform activities, such as walking, as well as the frequency with which these activities are performed. Therefore, parameters such as energy expenditure and the frequency and duration of particular physical activities are sensible outcome measures against which to judge the success of therapeutic interventions (Busse et al. 2004; Coleman et al. 1999).

Several approaches to the monitoring of different aspects of physical activities have recently been demonstrated. Among these approaches, both estimating metabolic energy expenditure and activity classification (see Mathie et al. 2004; Preece et al. 2008) from body-located accelerometer signals have shown great promise. A number of activity monitors are now available for lower limb activity monitoring (Godfrey et al. 2008). The reliability and validity of many of these monitors have been established (Grant et al. 2006; Haeuber et al. 2004; Resnick et al. 2001; Schasfoort et al. 2006; Welk et al. 2000).

4.3.3.4 Upper Limb Activity Monitors

In contrast to the trunk and lower limb, in which characteristic movements and postures are well defined (e.g. walking, sitting, lying), upper limb movements are considerably more varied. Despite these difficulties, a growing number of studies have recently investigated the possibility of upper limb activity monitoring.

Uswatte and colleagues (Uswatte et al. 2000) in a study of upper limb movement after a stroke, reported a system based on six accelerometers (two on each arm, one on the chest and one on the thigh of the affected side). The accelerometer output from the best four accelerometers was integrated over 2 s epochs and a fixed-threshold classifier used to classify data as corresponding to periods of arm movement, torso movement or walking (Uswatte et al. 2000). The results showed that it could correctly classify approximately 90% of epochs. Despite the limited nature of data obtained from this type of activity monitor, it has proved to be an objective and reliable measure to indicate the effectiveness of the rehabilitation programme in particular cases (Uswatte et al. 2000, 2005).

Schasfoort et al. (2003) reported the use of a complex system consisting of eight uniaxial accelerometers (one on each thigh, two on the chest, two on each wrist) originally developed by Tulen et al. (1997). The magnitude of the high pass filtered, rectified signal (corresponding to signal variability) was used to determine whether or not activity was taking place. Mean intensity of upper limb activity during sitting and standing; percentage of upper limb activity during sitting and standing, and; proportion of upper limb activity of one side relative to the other side, during sitting and standing, were reported.

Several studies have used the elevation of the arm as an indirect measure of activity. Vega-Gonzalez and colleagues (Vega-Gonzalez and Granat 2005) reported an upper limb activity monitor for an application similar to the work of Uswatte et al. (2000, 2005). This monitor used a pressure transducer attached to a length of fluid filled tubing running from the shoulder to the wrist. As the arm was raised, so the pressure increased and these data were logged over the course of the day. A threshold classifier allocated data to one of three categories: composite movement time, bimanual movement time, unimanual movement time. Similar studies, using multiple accelerometers to infer arm inclination and angular velocity have also been reported (e.g. Hansson et al. 2001; Bernmark and Wiktorin 2002).

The accuracy and between-day and between-subject variability of an inclinometer system were also evaluated (Hansson et al. 2001) where a previously developed inclinometer system (Hansson et al. 2006) was fixed on six healthy subjects, who were instructed to complete three work tasks. Based on at least three trials daily over seven days for each subject, the intra-subject variability was small but inter-subject variability was very large, suggesting that different individuals approach a given task in quite different but characteristic ways.

4.3.4 Activity Monitoring and Upper Limb Prosthesis Evaluation

Previous approaches to prosthetic evaluation have either quantified what a person can do in the laboratory or clinical environment, or used questionnaires/interviews that rely on self-reporting. Either can provide, at best, a gross approximation of aspects of prosthetic functional value.

New technology is emerging that makes the direct measurement of activity in daily life possible. However, the available upper limb activity monitors are limited in their outcomes and none is suitable for monitoring upper limb prostheses. Existing devices, many of which involve multiple accelerometers, estimate the frequency/magnitude of arm movements and the duration of arm movements. In some applications, such as regional pain syndrome (Schasfoort et al. 2006), movements of the upper limb cause pain and therefore patients tend to ignore the physical activities that require movement of the painful segments (Fordyce 1976; Jahanshahi and Philips 1986; Turk et al. 1985; Vlaeyen et al. 1987). Hence, detecting limb movements alone is a logical approach to the evaluation of the rehabilitation programme.

In the case of prosthetic evaluation, monitoring only the frequency and duration of arm movement is insufficient. Following a trans-radial amputation, amputees are normally able to move the residual limb freely. Further, the prosthetic device is intended to restore the functions of the wrist and hand. Therefore, simply identifying the presence or absence of movement of the upper limb does not indicate whether the prosthesis is used functionally or not.

It is proposed that an activity monitor for the upper limb prosthesis should enable identification of when the prosthesis is being used to perform functional tasks, a problem that cannot be directly inferred from hand opening data alone. The ability to identify the nature of the task being performed would allow for direct identification of the functional activities that the prosthetic user can or cannot perform and report the frequency of prosthesis use out of the view of clinical personnel. Thus, not only could the true functional loss of individuals be identified, and hence addressed by the rehabilitation programme, but designers of new prostheses would gain valuable insight into whether or not technical advances translated into benefit for the patient.

We present a new approach to upper limb activity monitoring that takes advantage of the particular characteristics of upper limb prostheses. Notably, we propose to monitor the opening/closing of the hand that must accompany the performance of a functional task. Such movements could easily be monitored using, for example, electrogoniometry or monitoring of the motor current in powered prosthetic hands. In so doing, we hope to be able to identify the period during which an object is being grasped (the so-called manipulation phase). Further, we propose the use of accelerometers to provide information on the orientation and acceleration of the prosthetic limb (and, if required, the non-amputated limb), which we hypothesise will contain information on the nature of the task being performed.

To detect the manipulation phase, and hence when to record acceleration signals, we presumed that the prosthetic hand remains closed (neutral position) when it is not in use and only opens when an object is going to be grasped or released. A simple state diagram illustrates the sequence of events associated with grasping and releasing an object (Fig. 4.5). Although this is arguably an oversimplification of what would happen in everyday life, it is a reasonable assumption for this feasibility study.

In the next section, we introduce a classifier that will use features of the pre-segmented acceleration signals to recognise the task and distinguish it from other functional and non-functional tasks. In so doing, it may be possible to monitor not

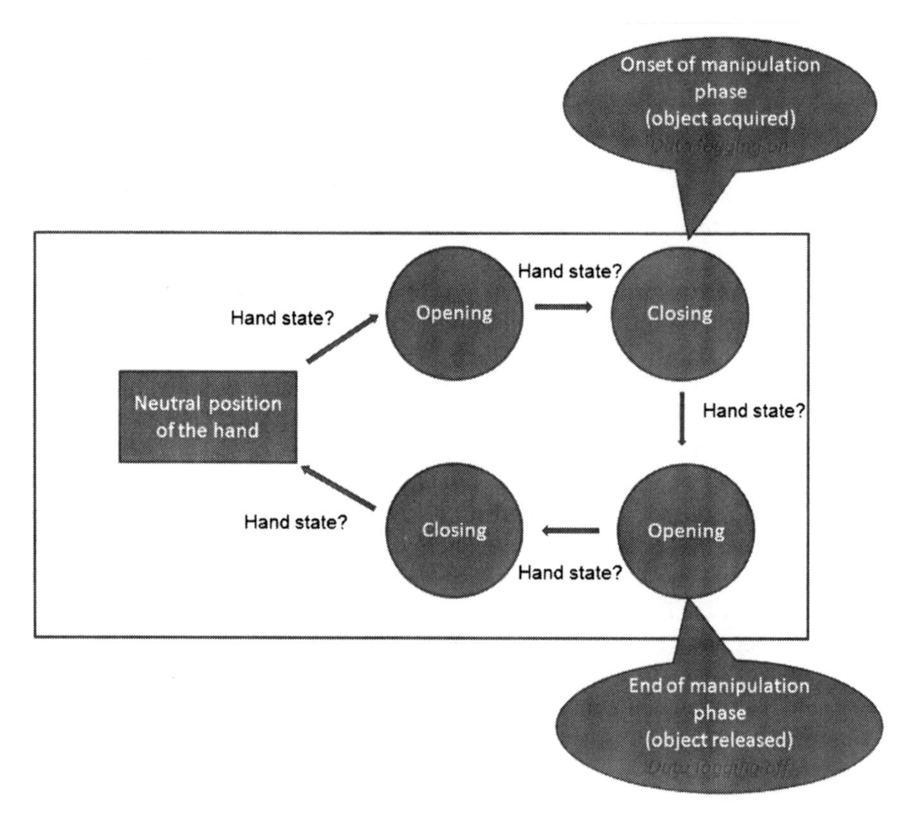

Fig. 4.5 State control to detect manipulation phase

only the presence or absence of upper limb activity, but potentially also the nature of the activity being performed.

Compared with the monitoring activities of the non-amputated upper limb, our approach is made potentially practical by the ease with which hand opening/closing may be monitored. Further characteristics that may make the problem of activity classification solvable in this case include:

- The reduced number of kinematic degrees of freedom of the prosthetic upper limb when compared with the anatomical limb;
- The observed tendency of amputees to perform upper limb tasks in a more repeatable manner than those with intact upper limbs (Black et al. 2005);
- The ability to locate accelerometers in a fixed position on the prosthetic forearm, thereby potentially reducing the day-to-day variations in sensor placement;
- The limited set of tasks that are reported to be performed by amputees using their prosthesis. Following unilateral upper limb amputation, the non-amputated side is reported to serve as the dominant side, irrespective of the situation prior to amputation (Fraser 1998; Thornby and Krebs 1992; van Lunteren et al. 1983), and the prosthesis is predominantly employed for performing bimanual tasks (Light et al. 2002; van Lunteren et al. 1983).

In Sect. 4.4, we report on the design of a case study to test whether our proposed approach is feasible and on the implementation of the classifier.

4.4 Methods

4.4.1 Introduction

In Sect. 4.3, we demonstrated the limitations with current approaches to prosthesis evaluation (questionnaires/interviews or laboratory-based studies) and introduced the concept of activity monitoring as a means of gathering information on both the type of activity being performed and the frequency with which it is carried out. We proposed a new activity monitoring approach that addresses the particular characteristics of trans-radial prostheses. In this section, we introduce an experimental design that we use to collect relevant motion data from two trans-radial myoelectric prosthesis users during the performance of a variety of tasks. We then describe the implementation of the approach introduced in Sect. 4.2.

The goal of this study was to identify whether it is possible to identify specific upper limb functional tasks (FTs) and specific upper limb non-functional tasks (NFTs), based only on information on the motion of limb segments and extent of hand opening. In this context, the FTs are defined as a set of bimanual tasks in which the prosthesis is actively used to grasp and release objects, and the NFTs as tasks that involve movement of the prosthesis but without active use of the prosthetic hand. We begin by describing the set of upper limb tasks and associated objects that we will use in our study.

4.4.1.1 Tasks and Objects Used in the Evaluation Study

In order to design the experimental work, a representative set of upper limb tasks and associated objects was required. As discussed earlier, it is well accepted that amputees rarely use their prosthetic hand to perform unilateral tasks (Black et al. 2005; Thornby and Krebs 1992; Light et al. 2002; van Lunteren et al. 1983) and hence we chose to focus on bimanual ADLs.

The manner in which tasks are performed with the prosthetic hand typically involves one hand serving as main manipulator (usually the non-amputated side) and the other as the stabiliser (usually the prosthetic side) (van Lunteren et al. 1983). van Lunteren et al. (1983) proposed that there are two basic approaches to object stabilisation: *active* in which the prosthesis is used to grasp and release objects; and *passive* in which the prosthesis does not grasp the object but is simply used to stabilise the object.

The argument for prescribing a myoelectric prosthesis is that it combines additional functionality with better cosmesis, when compared with the alternatives. Notably, active function is the only remarkable feature of this prosthesis. Therefore, in assessing the functionality that comes with a myoelectric prosthesis it is sensible to focus on tasks that require *active* involvement of the prosthesis.

In this work, a group of bimanual tasks used in previous direct-observation tests were considered for inclusion and only the subset of these that require active prosthetic use were selected for the experimental work (see Table 4.1). Since some of the tasks are commonly performed from both standing and sitting postures, these two postures were also included in the task definitions.

The set of different potential approaches to each task listed in Table 4.1 are described in Sobuh (2008). However, due to limited testing time it was not possible to include all of these approaches. A specific set of approaches to each task was selected by the first subject and the second subject was asked to use the same set.

The objects used for the selected bilateral tasks are shown in Fig. 4.6.

Table 4.1 The set of bimanual tasks (Y = yes, N = no)

Task description	Carried out from sitting posture	Carried out from standing posture
Simulating eating (Thornby & Krebs 1992, Bagley et al. 2006, Light et al. 2002, Wright et al. 2003)	Y	N
Opening a jar (Thornby & Krebs 1992)	Y	Y
Using a dustpan and a broom (Bagley et al. 2006)	N	Y
Pouring water into a glass (Weaver et al. 1988, Light et al. 2002)	Y	Y
Applying toothpaste to a toothbrush (Thornby & Krebs 1992)	N	Y

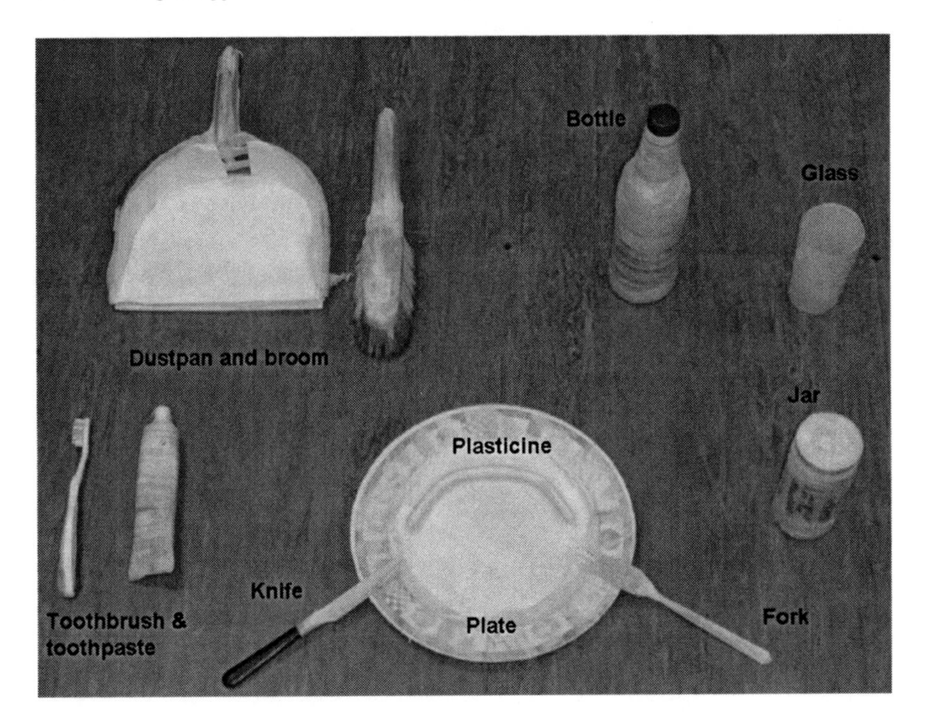

Fig. 4.6 Objects used in the experimental work

4.4.1.2 Final Experimental Design

The experiment consisted of two participants carrying out the set of FTs defined in Table 4.1 together with two common NFTs, namely arm swinging while walking and movement of the arm during the transition from walking to either sitting or standing.

One participant repeated the experiment on a different day. Figure 4.7 shows the sequence of events in the trials.

At this preliminary stage in the work it was decided to collect motion data from as many upper limb locations as was sensibly feasible and therefore instrumentation was placed on the prosthetic hand (measuring hand opening and wrist angle), both forearms and the non-amputated side upper arm to explore the effects of different sensor combinations on activity classification accuracy.

For this feasibility study, it was decided to use an optical motion capture system that allowed for position data on reflective markers located on the arm(s) and prosthetic index finger and thumb to be captured. On the basis of information, not only the acceleration of points on the arm but also the opening and closing of the hand, could be calculated. This approach allowed "virtual" accelerometers as well as "virtual" hand aperture sensors to be created, thus removing the need for any further instrumentation.

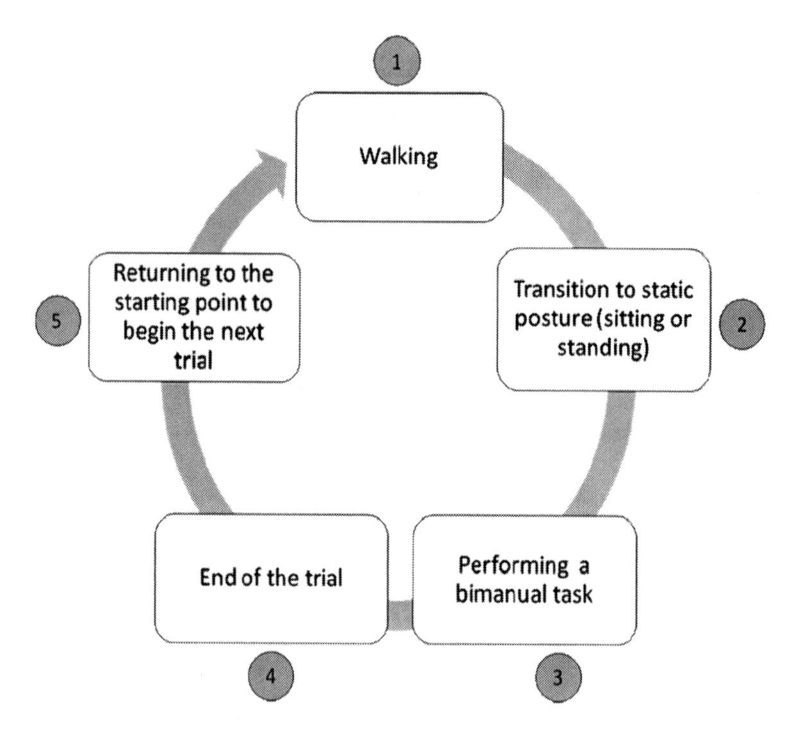

Fig. 4.7 The sequence of events in the laboratory trial

The experimental trials were conducted using a 10-camera motion capture system (Vicon 612® Vicon Motion Systems, Los Angeles, USA). The markers were located according to the CAST method (calibration anatomical systems technique) (Cappozzo et al. 1995, Cappozzo et al. 1996) and are shown in Fig. 4.8. Further details on the marker setup are available in Sobuh (2008).

4.4.1.3 Calculating Acceleration from Marker Data

Marker data were collected at 100 Hz and low-pass filtered with a fourth order Butterworth filter using a cutoff frequency of 6 Hz. The marker data were first passed to Vicon Workstation (Vicon Motion Systems, Los Angeles, USA) to label the data according to a previously defined kinematic model (Sobuh 2008). The labelled position data were then exported to a custom written programme developed from a software package, SMAS, developed previously by our group (Ren et al. 2005). SMAS was used to implement the filtering and to derive the linear acceleration of the marker clusters as well as the distance between the prosthetic index finger and prosthetic thumb. The calculation of linear acceleration from marker data used the approach described by Thies et al. (2007).

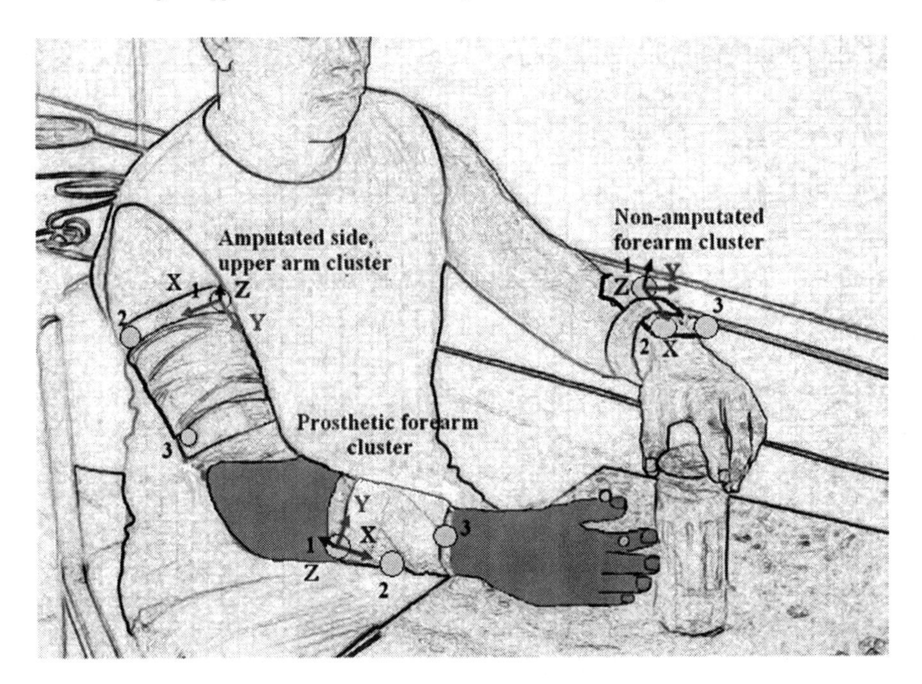

Fig. 4.8 Experimental setup. X axis was defined by the position data between markers 1 and 2, a temporary vector 't' was defined by the position data of markers 1 and 3, Z was defined by the cross product of X and t, and then the cross product of Z and X defined the Y axis

4.4.1.4 Subjects

Ethical approval for the study was obtained. The candidates were selected on the basis of following inclusion criteria:

1. Below elbow amputee;
2. Unilateral amputee;
3. Medically stable individual;
4. Residual limb 10 to 20 cm in length;
5. Stump in good general condition: absence of cuts, skin infection, excessive phantom pain, neuroma, bone prominence, and excessive perspiration;
6. No fixed contracture of the elbow;
7. No complications on the sound side;
8. No additional problems affecting the ability to reach and grasp, such as poor vision;
9. Fitted with a myoelectric prosthesis at least 1 year ago.

Two subjects were recruited to this case study (see Table 4.2). They were both considered successful users by their occupational therapists, and each wore a myoelectric prosthesis with a supracondylar socket, in which the suspension is achieved through location of the proximal contours of the socket over the epicondyles.

Table 4.2 The subjects

Subjects	Gender	Age	Height (cm)	Amputation side	Cause	Prosthesis
Subject 1	Male	38	176	Right	Tumour	Myoelectric Single-site-two-state
Subject 2	Male	42	180	Right	Traumatic injury	Myoelectric two-site-two-state

The second subject was also fitted with a figure-of-nine shoulder harness for additionally security.

4.4.1.5 Data Collection

Written consent was obtained from each subject prior to measurements being taken of upper limb range of motion and the shape of the residual limb.

Each subject was asked to adjust the table relative to the walkway to allow a smooth transition from walking to sitting. The subjects were then asked to complete the set of bimanual tasks (listed in Table 4.1) once prior to data collection, so they would be familiar with both the tasks and objects.

Each trial consisted of the subject walking from a start point along a 2 m path to a table, on which the objects to be grasped were located. The subject completed the particular bimanual task once (either from standing or sitting, as defined in Table 4.1). Once the ADL was completed, the subject walked back to the start point to get ready to commence the next trial. Each trial was repeated 15 times, making a total of 105 trials for each subject. The best 12 trials (those with the minimum number of marker occlusions) out of every 15 were considered for further analysis. This corresponded to 84 examples of walking, 48 examples of transition from walking to standing, 36 examples of transition from walking to sitting and 12 examples of each manipulation phase.

The second subject visited the lab for a re-test almost 1 year after the first test. Between the first and second tests, the subject had been fitted with a new myoelectric prosthesis. The new prosthesis incorporated a very similar hand and used the same control strategy as the previous one, used a similar socket, but did not require the use of a shoulder harness. Table 4.3 lists the approaches that were used to complete the tasks in the study.

4.4.1.6 Data Structure and Segmentation

In this study, we constrained both the set of phases and the sequence in which they took place (as shown in Fig. 4.9 below). We chose to segment the data based on a combination of observation of hand opening data and other marker data, using a purpose written software tool written for the purpose, the Eventlabeller, Fig. 4.10.

The Eventlabeller provides a simple approach to segmenting the data. The data sets are imported and displayed in the bottom right corner of the Eventlabeller.

Table 4.3 The tasks and their performed approaches

Task description	The performed approaches
Simulating eating	The fork is handed to the prosthesis by the subject's non-amputated hand, and then the knife is held by the non-amputated hand. The piece of plasticine is fixed by the fork and the knife is used to cut the plasticine
Opening a jar (from sitting)	The jar is stabilised against the table by the prosthetic hand and the lid is removed by the non-amputated hand
Opening a jar (from standing)	The jar is handed to the prosthetic hand by the non-amputated hand, and then the lid is removed by the non-amputated hand
Using a dustpan and a broom	The dustpan is handed to the prosthetic hand by the non-amputated hand, then the broom is held by the non-amputated hand, after which the dustpan is directed toward the broom which is used to sweep the surface
Pouring water into a glass (from sitting)	The glass is handed to the prosthetic hand by the non-amputated hand then the bottle is held by the non-amputated hand and while the glass is being held securely by the prosthetic hand in the air, water is poured from the bottle
Pouring water into a glass (from standing)	The glass is handed to the prosthetic hand by the non-amputated hand then the bottle is held by the non-amputated hand and while the glass is being held securely by the prosthetic hand in the air, water is poured from the bottle
Applying toothpaste to a toothbrush	The brush is handed to the prosthetic hand by the non-amputated hand, and the toothpaste is held by the non-amputated hand and then applied to the brush

When a trial is selected, the acceleration signals calculated from the marker cluster position data, in addition to the distance between the index and thumb of the prosthetic hand, are displayed in a window at the middle of the Eventlabeller.

To define the start and end of walking, transition and manipulation phases from data collected in a single trial, the motion of the markers throughout the trial is viewed in the "Task viewer". The "movement controllers" allow the user to move forward or backward in time. Based on visual inspection of the data, the "class controller" allows the user to label the frame numbers associated with transition between phases. Once labelling is complete, the labelled data are exported to file.

4.4.1.7 Activity Classification

The goal of the work, as mentioned earlier, was to identify whether or not it was feasible to use accelerometer outputs derived from the motion of limb segments, appropriately segmented using a measure of the prosthetic hand opening, to identify the functional upper limb tasks and distinguish them from other non-functional tasks.

Many different analytical approaches have been developed and used for such a classification problem (see for example Chau (2001a, b), Preece et al. (2008)). Chau attempts to establish general guidelines for selecting an appropriate analytical

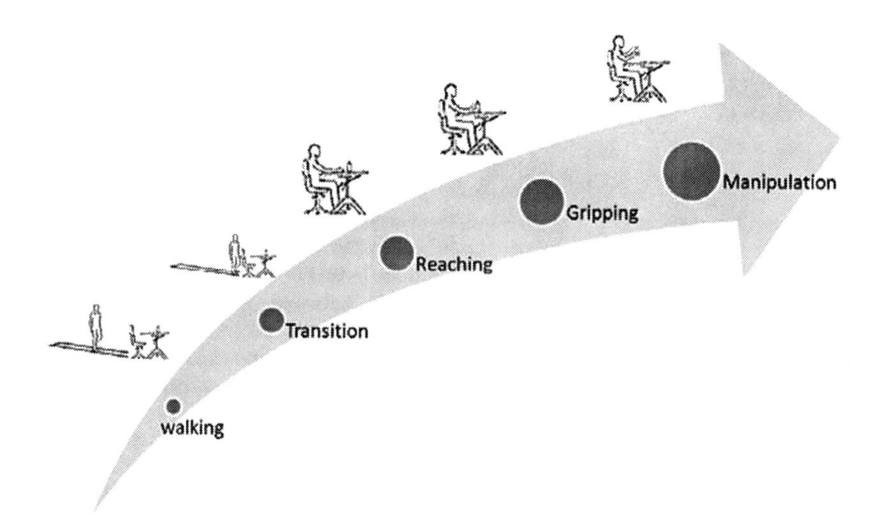

Fig. 4.9 Sequence of phases within a single trial. The figure shows one example of a task (performed from sitting). However, tasks performed from standing exhibit the same sequence

method for a given specific purpose, comparing and recommending a number of approaches based on their applicability under different scenarios. In the case of the lower limb, it was reported that Artificial Neural Networks (ANNs) are widely used for classification problems (Chau 2001a). We therefore adopt the ANN approach for the upper limb because the upper limb and lower limb motion data share many common features. However, we also note that the upper limb is more extreme in the sense that it is more mobile and less constrained than the lower limb.

ANNs are mathematical models (Bishop 2005) originally inspired by the function of biological neurons but later placed on a solid statistical foundation. An ANN is composed of simple elements (nodes or units), functioning simultaneously and in parallel, whose interaction (via connections with associated weights) generates a vector of output values (Fig. 4.11).

ANNs provide a flexible means of "learning" complex relationships within data sets without making assumptions about the specific nature of any relationship. This is achieved by adjusting the parameters (i.e. weights) of the network in such a way as to minimise the error between the predicted output and actual (or target) output in response to a set of input patterns (training data). They have proven very popular due to properties such as tolerance to noisy training data (by modelling the conditional mean of the output distribution) and automatic relevance determination for identifying redundant training data (Bishop 2005). For this feasibility work, the popular feedforward multi-layer perceptron (MLP) neural network with a single hidden layer was used as the classifier, as is used in many other applications (Chau 2001a).

In order to demonstrate the feasibility of the approach, the classifier was trained and tested using a number of pre-segmented data sets that corresponded to the manipulation, walking and transition data from each of the trials.

Since each example consists of a large (and varying) number of samples, the raw acceleration data was not suitable as an input pattern for the ANN. Therefore, each

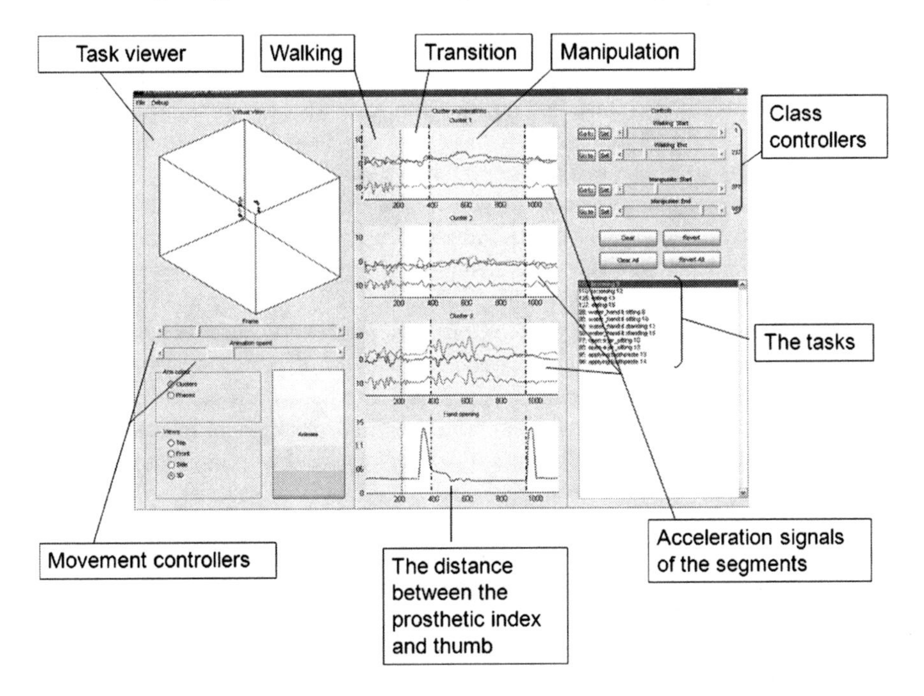

Fig. 4.10 The Eventlabeller

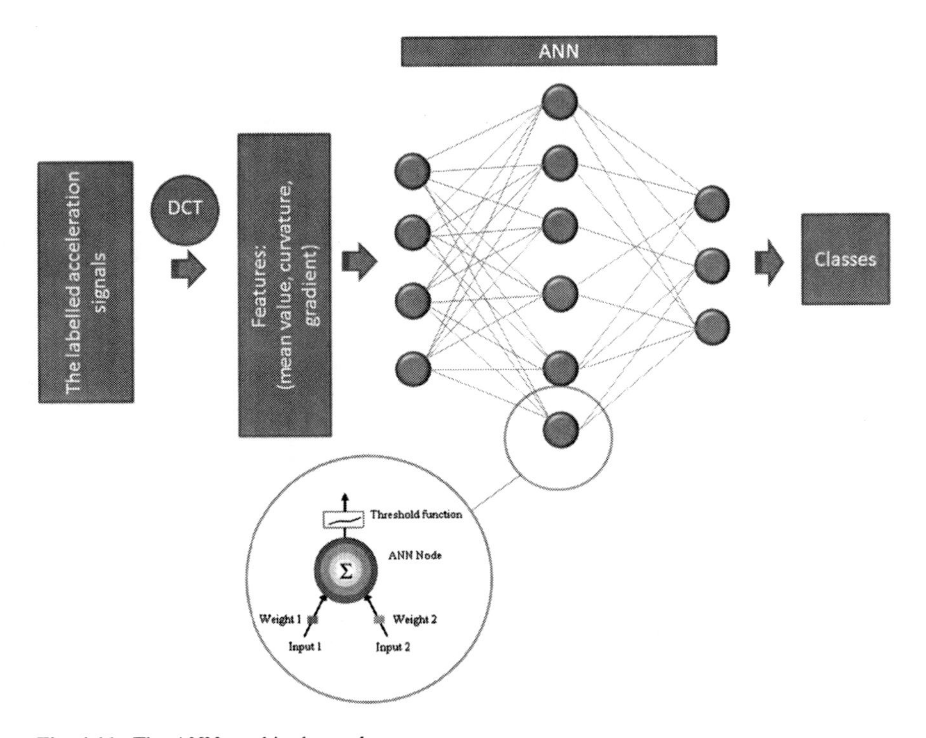

Fig. 4.11 The ANN used in the study

signal was first pre-processed in order to reduce it to a low-dimensional feature vector that retained the most important signal properties. Specifically, the discrete cosine transform (DCT) (Chau 2001a) was computed for each signal in each of the three axes (*X*, *Y* and *Z*) and the first three coefficients – corresponding approximately to mean value, gradient and curvature – used to build a feature vector.

In order to evaluate the performance of the ANN for activity classification within subject, a "leave-one-out" training/testing technique was applied. In this technique, a single sample is omitted from the complete data set and the classifier is optimised with the remaining training samples. The error of the classifier is then recorded when tested on the removed sample. Repeating this for every sample and computing the average error gives a robust estimate of performance that is not dependent on the particular training/testing split. For the within subject testing, we defined a sample as the feature vector corresponding to a single trial that comprised a walking, a transition (either standing or sitting) and a manipulation phase. The average classification accuracy was calculated for both subjects.

The performance of the ANN for activity classification between subjects was also explored. In this case, the training data includes all examples from one subject, whereas the testing data included all examples from the other subject. The training/testing order is then reversed and the average classification accuracy calculated.

Furthermore, the stability of the ANN performance over time was estimated on one subject (test and retest reliability). This was applied by training the ANN using all data collected on one day and testing it using all data collected on a second day. The training/testing order was then reversed and the average classification accuracy calculated.

Finally, we reduced the complexity of the classification task by considering the set of tasks to belong to one of two classes, either FTs or NFTs. The classifier's ability to distinguish between these two classes was tested between days.

4.5 Results

4.5.1 Subjects and Data

Two subjects (1, 2) completed testing on one day; subject 2 also completed the tests on a second day. Each subject at each visit completed the 105 trials, as described in Sect. 4.4.1.5.

The collected data were digitised, smoothed and used to calculate accelerations at the centres of the marker clusters (referred to from this point on as "virtual sensors") of interest. For each trial the manipulation phase of each task together with data collected during both walking and transition phases were labelled using the Eventlabeller.

Some examples of labelled acceleration data from the virtual sensor on the prosthesis for both subjects are shown in Fig. 4.12 (each trial is normalised to 500 samples, for ease of comparison).

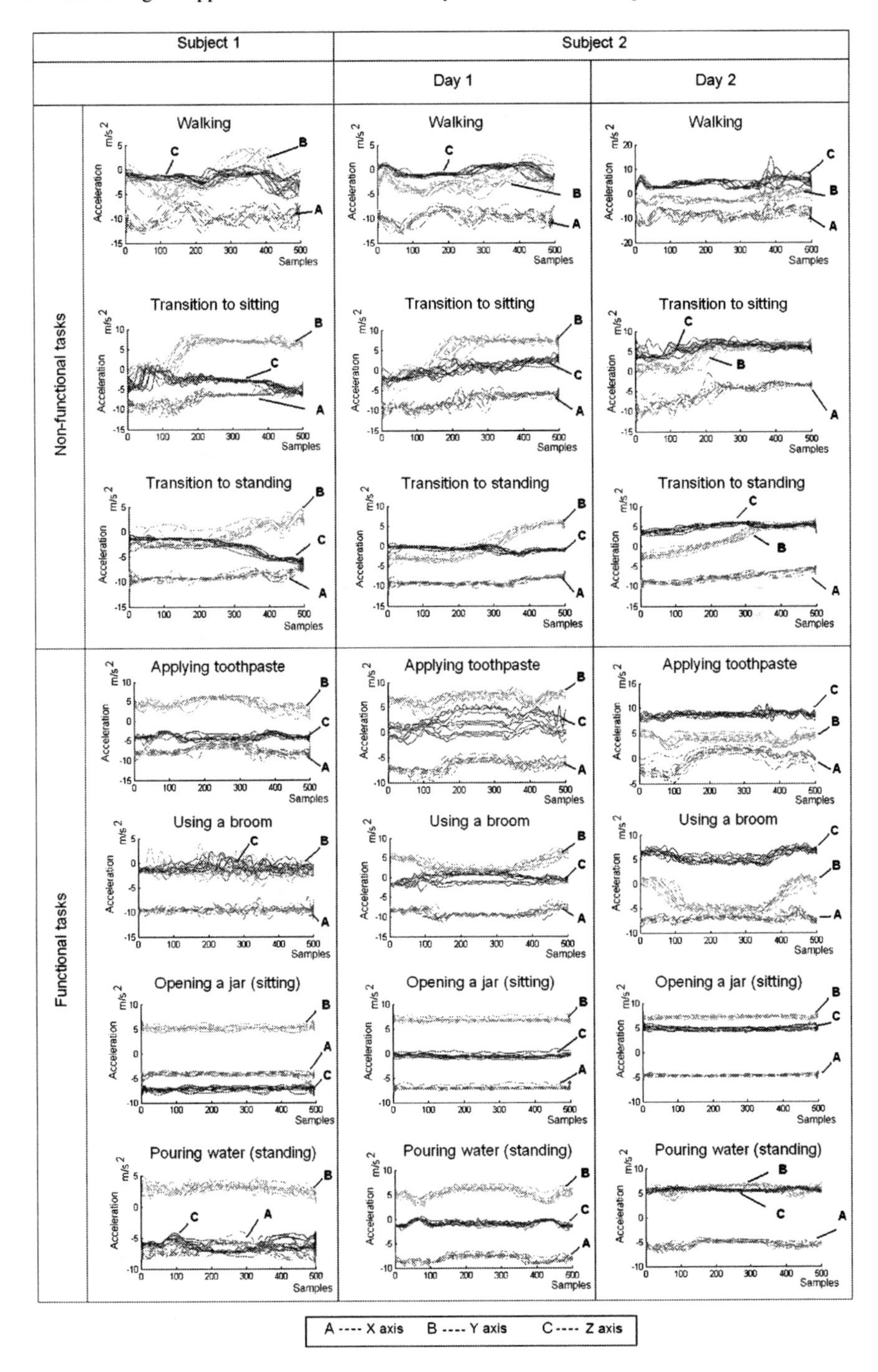

Fig. 4.12 Examples of the labelled acceleration waveforms of subject 1, subject 2 and subject 2 (day 2) (data of the prosthetic forearm virtual sensor)

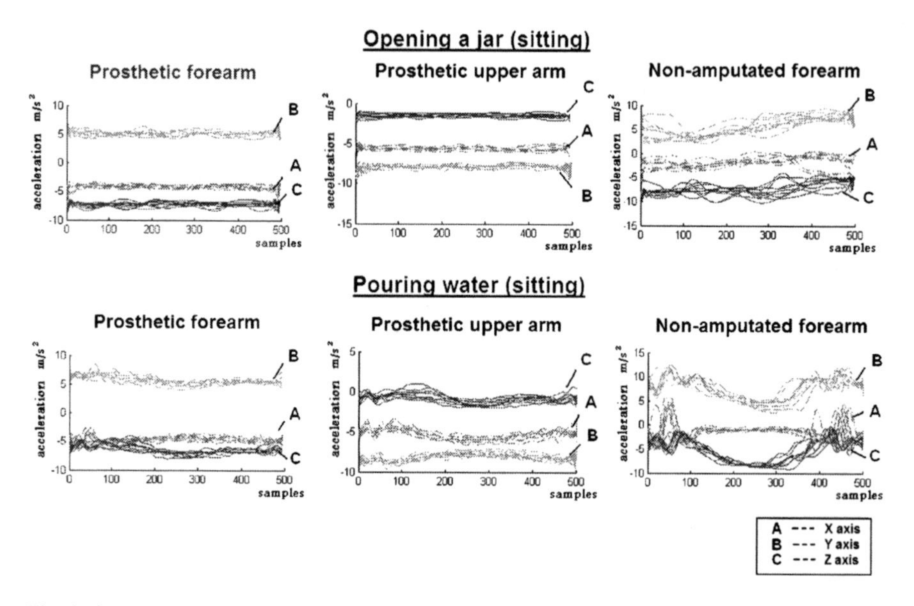

Fig. 4.13 Acceleration waveforms for subject 1 from 3 different limb locations during performance of two different tasks "open a jar (sitting)" (*top*) and "pour water (sitting)" (*bottom*)

Figure 4.13 shows an example of data from the three virtual sensors of interest (prosthetic forearm, prosthetic side upper arm and non-amputated forearm).

4.5.2 The Neural Network and Task Classification

This section reports the results of task classification using the ANN (more specifically MLP) based on the acceleration signals gathered during the manipulation phase of the tasks and during walking and transition phases. The classification was assumed to be 100% successful if the ANN was able to correctly identify the tasks associated with the manipulation phase data and the different non-functional tasks, walking and transition.

The classification performance of the ANN was first assessed within and between subjects as well as between days, based on acceleration data derived from the virtual sensors on the upper and forearm on the prosthetic side and the non-amputated forearm. Finally, the effects on classification accuracy of reducing the virtual sensor set were explored by considering the following four conditions:

Condition 1: All three virtual sensors (prosthetic forearm, prosthetic upper arm and non-amputated forearm) were included in the classification;

Condition 2: Both prosthetic forearm virtual sensor data and the non-amputated forearm virtual sensor data were included;

Condition 3: Both prosthetic forearm virtual sensor data and the amputated side upper arm virtual sensor data were included;

Condition 4: Only data from the prosthetic forearm virtual sensor were included.

Within subject classification was carried out using a "leave-one-out" training/testing technique. Interestingly, the ANN exhibited 100% within subject classification accuracy within day, as all tasks (functional and non-functional) performed by subjects 1 and 2 were classified correctly for conditions 1 and 2. This was reduced only slightly to 99.4% accuracy for conditions 3 and 4 (Fig. 4.14).

Between subjects classification accuracy was also estimated. Depending on the number of virtual sensors used, accuracy ranged between 81% and 91.9% (Fig. 4.14).

When assessing the stability of the ANN performance *between days,* accuracy ranged between 84% and 98% (Fig. 4.14), depending on the number of virtual sensors used.

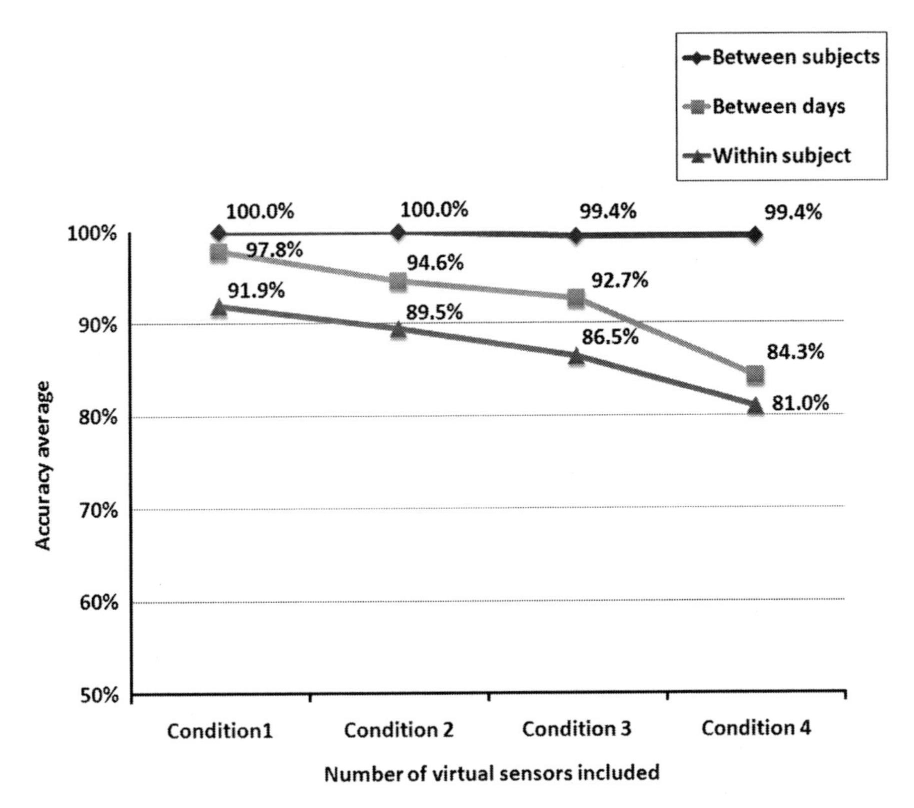

Fig. 4.14 Average classification accuracy within and between subjects and days with four different virtual sensor sets

To illustrate in more detail the specific types of misclassification that occurred, Table 4.4 shows an example of the resulting confusion matrix for between subjects training/testing (using data of both prosthetic and non-amputated forearm sensors).

Finally, the ability of the ANN to differentiate between functional and non-functional tasks was investigated between days. The investigation was carried out first using all virtual sensor data, and then the three other reduced virtual sensor sets (as described above). It was found that the ANN was 100% accurate when data from all virtual sensors were used, and dropped to 99%, 98% and 93% for the three other conditions respectively.

Figure 4.14 highlights the effect of virtual sensor reduction on within subject, between subjects and between days classification accuracy.

4.6 Discussion and Conclusions

4.6.1 Discussion

In this study, we have demonstrated the feasibility of monitoring upper limb prosthesis activity. A methodology has been presented that allows for rapid collection of simulated hand state and accelerometer data from upper limb amputees during walking, transition and while performing appropriate bimanual tasks. Data collected during the trials were pre-processed using a bespoke tool, the Eventlabeller, which was used to label data corresponding to a range of functional and non-functional tasks. Based on the labelled 3D simulated acceleration signals from the upper limbs, an ANN was trained to classify the data. *Within subject, between subjects and between days* classification accuracy using acceleration data from all arm locations were investigated as well as the effects on classification of reducing the virtual sensor set.

Although, in this study, the data were pre-segmented using the Eventlabeller tool before being supplied to the ANN, a practical implementation of our approach would use hand opening/closing events to segment the data. As these events, although likely to correspond to functional task performance, may also occur during the performance of non-functional tasks, such as walking, we investigated the ability of the classifier to distinguish between such data sets.

The result of the case study with two subjects has allowed us to draw provisional conclusions regarding the feasibility of an upper limb activity monitoring system.

4.6.1.1 Subject-Specific or Generalised Neural Network?

As illustrated in Fig. 4.12, acceleration data characterising upper limb motion during a range of tasks, when collected under controlled conditions, appear to be reasonably repeatable *within subject and within day. Between subject data* exhibit

Table 4.4 A confusion matrix of the between-days ANN testing result (virtual sensors on both prosthetic and non-amputated forearms)*

Classes	Walking	Transition to standing	Transition to sitting	Applying toothpaste	Using a broom	Simulating eating	Opening a jar (sitting)	Open a jar (standing)	Pouring water (sitting)	Pouring water (standing)
Walking	82	0	0	1	0	0	0	0	0	1
Transition to standing	0	48	0	0	0	0	0	0	0	0
Transition to sitting	0	0	36	0	0	0	0	0	0	0
Applying toothpaste	0	0	0	8	0	0	3	0	0	0
Using a broom	9	0	0	0	0	0	3	0	0	0
Simulating eating	0	0	0	0	0	12	0	0	0	0
Open a jar (sitting)	0	0	0	0	0	0	8	0	4	0
Open a jar (standing)	0	0	0	0	0	0	1	11	0	0
Pouring water (sitting)	0	0	0	0	0	0	0	0	12	0
Pouring water (standing)	0	0	0	3	0	0	1	0	0	8

*In the confusion matrix, figures running diagonally (from the upper left corner to the lower right one) indicate how many times the ANN classified the tasks correctly (e.g. 82 times for walking). The off-diagonal figures refer to the number of times the ANN misclassified the tasks (e.g. twice for walking: once recognised as applying toothpaste and once recognised as pouring water (standing)) qualitatively different characteristic curves (Fig. 4.12). These observations are supported by considering the classification results which suggest that, for a particular individual, the activities are well-separated in feature space.

As can be seen from Fig. 4.14, even using data from all virtual sensor locations, the *between subject* accuracy drops from 100% to just over 90%. With the minimum virtual sensor set (single 3D accelerometer mounted on the prosthesis socket, plus hand opening detection system), the accuracy is observed to drop to just over 80%. It is therefore assumed that a future implementation of our approach would most likely be based on an ANN *customised for each user*. Accordingly, the following paragraphs discuss the classification results obtained from within subjects and between days training/testing only.

4.6.1.2 Between Day Performance

Although the acceleration data of manipulation phases (see Figs. 4.12 and 4.13) show some clear changes over time, this may be partly an artefact resulting from changes in cluster location on the prosthetic forearm between days 1 and 2 and also influenced by the change in prosthesis between visits. However, the changes, even over almost a year, did not dramatically affect the classification accuracy of the ANN. This suggests that the proposed monitoring approach, based on the use of an individually trained ANN, may be feasible for both short and long term monitoring applications.

4.6.1.3 Data from Single or Multiple Locations on the Body?

As can be seen from Fig. 4.12, acceleration data calculated from the virtual sensor on the prosthesis generally provided qualitatively different characteristic curves across the different tasks. For tasks where the prosthetic limb remains relatively stationary, such as “open a jar (sitting)” and “pour water (sitting)”, unsurprisingly there is little observable difference between the two subsets. However, as can be seen from Fig. 4.13, accelerations recorded of the other upper limb segments, and particularly, of the non-amputated forearm, show much more distinct differences between the two subsets. Therefore, as the results in Fig. 4.14 indicate, the overall classification accuracy is improved if acceleration data from two or more virtual sensors are fed into the ANN; in particular data of the prosthesis virtual sensor and non-amputated forearm.

4.6.1.4 Functional vs. Non-functional Tasks

At the most general level of task classification, upper limb activities can considered as either functional or non-functional. In the context of upper limb prosthesis monitoring, this level of classification would allow the clinician or designer to conclude as to the extent to which a prosthesis is functionally used.

As shown earlier in Sect. 4.5, the ANN misclassified functional as non-functional tasks (and vice versa) only a small number of times. This was still the case even when data calculated from the virtual sensor on the prosthetic forearm was used for the classification (93% average accuracy). This suggested that data obtained from one virtual sensor on the prosthesis, together with information about the hand status, would provide a quantitative approach to evaluate general prosthetic usage (i.e. the number of hours/day that the prosthesis was used to perform functional tasks).

4.6.2 Future Work

The work presented here has described a new approach to upper limb activity monitoring in upper limb amputees based on acceleration data. The initial results suggest that our approach has the potential to be used in a future practical system. However, there remains further work to be carried out before a conclusive answer to the question of feasibility of upper limb activity monitoring in amputees can be obtained.

In the first place, the protocol needs to be tested/retested on a larger population and should include a larger number of tasks. Such a study should be performed with a less constrained set of tasks, in which the subjects can choose the manner in which the tasks are carried out. Furthermore, although the simulated accelerometer data shows good correspondence with physical accelerometer data (Thies et al. 2007) the effect on classification accuracy has yet to be tested. Nevertheless, based on the features implemented in this study, it is unlikely that any significant differences between the feature values would be observed and hence the impact would be low.

Another question remaining is the extent to which the data could be segmented on the basis of hand opening/closing. Although it is thought that users would tend to keep the hand at a fixed aperture between periods of functional task performance, this has yet to be established outside of the laboratory and further work would be required to investigate this element. Clearly, such a study can only take place once a system for monitoring hand state is implemented.

Although the implemented ANN was customised for this work, its settings were not optimised. For instance, the ANN carries out classification on the basis of "features" derived from the input signals (acceleration waveforms in this case). In this work, objects were pragmatically characterised by three features (mean value, gradient and curvature) derived from the discrete cosine transform. Alternative ways of characterising the waveforms could lead to improved classification accuracy.

As linear acceleration on a rigid body that is both translating and rotating (the general case of the prosthesis) is location dependent, the signal measured by an accelerometer will depend on its location on the prosthesis. One of the future objectives is to define the optimal limb locations on which the best discriminative acceleration signals, and thus the best classification accuracy, can be obtained. With the approach demonstrated in this work, together with a simple model of the geometry of the prosthesis, it would be possible to simulate the outputs from accelerometers located at a number of different locations on the prosthesis and explore the effect these may have on classification accuracy. This approach has recently been demonstrated for the upper limb application by the Salford team (Tresadern et al. 2009).

4.7 Conclusion

This study represents the first attempt to systematically describe and analyse prosthetic upper limb motion while performing bimanual tasks on the basis of the limbs' acceleration. A detailed protocol for tracking and analysing upper limb motion in the movement laboratory has been established. A practical, yet justifiable, set of tasks to be used in the experiments has been proposed and integrated into a protocol, including sequences of walking and bimanual task completion. Using the prosthetic hand state as a marker, the manipulation phase has been reliably identified, which will be a critical element in any future activity monitoring system.

Finally, an approach to classifying the tasks using an ANN has been demonstrated. The results revealed that the ANN could accurately discriminate between functional and non-functional tasks using acceleration data from the manipulation phase on the basis of only one virtual sensor (93% accuracy between days when only the data of the prosthesis marker cluster was employed). Furthermore, using acceleration data of two virtual sensors (on both forearms) the ANN was shown to be able to discriminate between the nature of the functional tasks being performed with 95% accuracy. The ANN performance was found to be generally stable over time. The results, although only demonstrated on case studies, provide strong support for further work.

Acknowledgements The authors gratefully acknowledge the financial support from the University of Jordan and thank the participants in the study. The authors also acknowledge colleagues at the University of Strathclyde for their assistance with figures 4.2–4.4.

References

Agnew PJ (1981) Functional effectiveness of a myo-electric prosthesis compared with a functional split-hook prosthesis: a single subject experiment. Prosthet Orthot Int 5:2–96

Bagley AM, Molitor F, Wagner LV et al (2006) The unilateral below elbow test: a function test for children with unilateral congenital below elbow deficiency. Dev Med Child Neurol 48:569–575

Bergman K, Ornholmer L, Zackrisson K et al (1992) Functional benefit of an adaptive myoelectric prosthetic hand compared to a conventional myoelectric hand. Prosthet Orthot Int 16:32–37

Bernmark E, Wiktorin C (2002) A triaxial accelerometer for measuring arm movements. Appl Ergon 33:541–547

Bishop CM (2005) Neural networks for pattern recognition. Oxford university press, Oxford, UK

Black N, Biden EN, Rickards J (2005) Using potential energy to measure work related activities for persons wearing upper limb prostheses. Robotica 23:319–327
Buffart LM, Roebroeck ME, Pesch-Batenburg JM et al (2006) Assessment of arm/hand functioning in children with a congenital transverse or longitudinal reduction deficiency of the upper limb. Disabil Rehabil 28:85–95
Burger H, Marincek C (1994) Upper limb prosthetic use in Slovenia. Prosthet Orthot Int 18:25–33
Burger H, Brezovar D, Marincek C (2004) Comparison of clinical test and questionnaires for the evaluation of upper limb prosthetic use in children. Disabil Rehabil 26:911–916
Busse ME, Pearson OR, Van Deursen R et al (2004) Quantified measurement of activity provides insight into motor function and recovery in neurological disease. J Neurol Neurosurg Psychiatry 75:884–888
Bussmann HB, Reuvekamp PJ, Veltink PH et al (1998) Validity and reliability of measurements obtained with an "activity monitor" in people with and without a transtibial amputation. Phys Ther 78:989–998
Cappozzo A, Catani F, Croce UD, et al (1995) Position and orientation in space of bones during movement: anatomical frame definition and determination. Clin Biomech (Bristol, Avon) 10:171–178
Cappozzo A, Catani F, Leardini A et al (1996) Position and orientation in space of bones during movement: experimental artefacts. Clin Biomech (Bristol, Avon) 11:90–100
Chau T (2001a) A review of analytical techniques for gait data. Part 2: neural network and wavelet methods. Gait Posture 13:102–120
Chau T (2001b) A review of analytical techniques for gait data. Part 1: fuzzy, statistical and fractal methods. Gait Posture 13:49–66
Coleman KL, Smith DG, Boone DA et al (1999) Step activity monitor: long-term, continuous recording of ambulatory function. J Rehabil Res Dev 36:8–18
Culhane KM, O'Connor M, Lyons D et al (2005) Accelerometers in rehabilitation medicine for older adults. Age Ageing 34:556–560
Edelstein JE, Berger N (1993) Performance comparison among children fitted with myoelectric and body-powered hands. Arch Phys Med Rehabil 74:376–380
Fordyce W (1976) Behavioral methods for chronic pain and illness. Mosby, St. Louis, MO
Fraser CM (1998) An evaluation of the use made of cosmetic and functional prostheses by unilateral upper limb amputees. Prosthet Orthot Int 22:216–223
Gaine WJ, Smart C, Bransby-Zachary M (1997) Upper limb traumatic amputees. Review of prosthetic use. J Hand Surg [Br] 22:73–76
Gambrell CR (2008) Overuse syndrome and the unilateral upper limb amputee: consequences and prevention. J Prosthet Orthot 20:126
Godfrey A, Conway R, Meagher D et al (2008) Direct measurement of human movement by accelerometry. Med Eng Phys 30:1364–1386
Grant PM, Ryan CG, Tigbe WW et al (2006) The validation of a novel activity monitor in the measurement of posture and motion during everyday activities. Br J Sports Med 40:992–997
Haeuber E, Shaughnessy M, Forrester LW et al (2004) Accelerometer monitoring of home- and community-based ambulatory activity after stroke. Arch Phys Med Rehabil 85:1997–2001
Hansson G, Asterland P, Holmer N et al (2001) Validity and reliability of triaxial accelerometers for inclinometry in posture analysis. Med Biol Eng Comput 39:405–413
Hansson GA, Arvidsson I, Ohlsson K et al (2006) Precision of measurements of physical workload during standardised manual handling. Part II: Inclinometry of head, upper back, neck and upper arms. J Electromyogr Kinesiol 16:125–136
Hermansson LM, Fisher AG, Bernspang B et al (2005) Assessment of capacity for myoelectric control: a new Rasch-built measure of prosthetic hand control. J Rehabil Med 37:166–171
Hermansson LM, Bodin L, Eliasson AC (2006) Intra- and inter-rater reliability of the assessment of capacity for myoelectric control. J Rehabil Med 38:118–123
Jahanshahi M, Philips C (1986) Validating a new technique for the assessment of pain behaviour. Behav Res Ther 24:35–42

Jones LE, Davidson JH (1999) Save that arm: a study of problems in the remaining arm of unilateral upper limb amputees. Prosthet Orthot Int 23:55–58

Kejlaa GH (1993) Consumer concerns and the functional value of prostheses to upper limb amputees. Prosthet Orthot Int 17:157–163

Light CM, Chappell PH, Kyberd PJ et al (1999) A critical review of functionality assessment of natural and prosthetic hands. Br J Occup Ther 62:7–12

Light CM, Chappell PH, Kyberd PJ (2002) Establishing a standardized clinical assessment tool of pathologic and prosthetic hand function: Normative data, reliability, and validity. Arch Phys Med Rehabil 83:776–783

Malone JM, Fleming LL, Roberson J et al (1984) Immediate, early, and late postsurgical management of upper-limb amputation. J Rehabil Res Dev 21:33–41

Mathie MJ, Coster ACF, Lovell NH et al (2004) Accelerometry: providing an integrated, practical method for long-term, ambulatory monitoring of human movement. Physiol Meas 25:R1–R20

Meier RH, Atkins DJ (2004) Functional restoration of adults and children with upper extremity amputation. Demos, New York

Millstein SG, Heger H, Hunter GA (1986) Prosthetic use in adult upper limb amputees: a comparison of the body powered and electrically powered prostheses. Prosthet Orthot Int 10:27–34

Muzumdar A (2004) Powered upper limb prostheses: control, implementation and clinical application. Springer, Berlin

NASDAB (2005) The amputee statistical database for the United Kingdom [annual report] (2005/06) Information Services Division, NHS Scotland. Edinburgh. http://www.nasdab.co.uk/pdf.pl?file=nasdab/news/080117_(web)_CompleteReport.pdf. Accessed 28 Dec 2008

Northmore-Ball MD, Heger H, Hunter GA (1980) The below-elbow myo-electric prosthesis. A comparison of the Otto Bock myo-electric prosthesis with the hook and functional hand. J Bone Joint Surg Br 62:363–367

Pezzin LE, Dillingham TR, Mackenzie EJ et al (2004) Use and satisfaction with prosthetic limb devices and related services. Arch Phys Med Rehabil 85:723–729

Preece SJ, Goulermas JY, Kenney LP, Howard D, Meijer K, Crompton R. (2009) Activity identification using body-mounted sensors – A review of classification techniques. Physiol Meas. 30(4):R1–33

Pruitt SD, Varni JW, Setoguchi Y (1996) Functional status in children with limb deficiency: development and initial validation of an outcome measure. Arch Phys Med Rehabil 77:1233–1238

Pruitt SD, Varni JW, Seid M et al (1998) Functional status in limb deficiency: development of an outcome measure for preschool children. Arch Phys Med Rehabil 79:405–411

Pruitt SD, Seid M, Varni JW et al (1999) Toddlers with limb deficiency: conceptual basis and initial application of a functional status outcome measure. Arch Phys Med Rehabil 80:819–824

Ren L, Jones R, Howard D (2005) A software package for three-dimensional motion analysis of general biomechanical multi-body systems. In: Proceedings of biomechanics of the lower limb in health, disease and rehabilitation, University of Salford, UK, 122–123

Resnick B, Nahm ES, Orwig D et al (2001) Measurement of activity in older adults: reliability and validity of the step activity monitor. J Nurs Meas 9:275–290

Roeschlein RA, Domholdt E (1989) Factors related to successful upper extremity prosthetic use. Prosthet Orthot Int 13:14–18

Schasfoort FC, Bussmann JB, Zandbergen AM et al (2003) Impact of upper limb complex regional pain syndrome type 1 on everyday life measured with a novel upper limb-activity monitor. Pain 101:79–88

Schasfoort FC, Bussmann JB, Krijnen HJ et al (2006) Upper limb activity over time in complex regional pain syndrome type 1 as objectively measured with an upper limb-activity monitor: an explorative multiple case study. Eur J Pain 10:31–39

Silcox DH, Rooks MD, Vogel RR et al (1993) Myoelectric prostheses. A long-term follow-up and a study of the use of alternate prostheses. J Bone Joint Surg Am 75:1781–1789

Smith DG, Michael JW, Bowker JH (2004) Atlas of amputations and limb deficiencies: Surgical, prosthetic, and rehabilitation principles. American Academy of Orthopaedic Surgeons, Rosemont, IL

Sobuh M (2008) Monitoring of upper limb prosthesis activity in trans-radial amputees – A feasibility study. MSc thesis Institute for Health & Social Care Research (IHSCR), School of Health Care Professions. University of Salford, Salford, UK

Tresadern PA, Thies SB, Kenney LP, Howard D, Smith C, Rigby J, Goulermas JY (2009) Simulating acceleration from stereophotogrammetry for medical device design. J Biomech Eng 131(6):061002

Thies SB, Tresadern P, Kenney L et al (2007) Comparison of linear accelerations from three measurement systems during "reach & grasp". Med Eng Phys 29:967–972

Thornby MA, Krebs DE (1992) Bimanual skill development in pediatric below-elbow amputation: a multicenter, cross-sectional study. Arch Phys Med Rehabil 73:697–702

Tulen JH, Bussmann HB, van Steenis HG et al (1997) A novel tool to quantify physical activities: ambulatory accelerometry in psychopharmacology. J Clin Psychopharmacol 17:202–207

Turk DC, Wack JT, Kerns RD (1985) An empirical examination of the "pain-behavior" construct. J Behav Med 8:119–130

UNB test of prosthetics function: A test for unilateral upper extremity amputees, ages 2-13 [test manual] (1985) Bio-Engineering Institute, University of Brunswick. Fredericton, New Brunswick. http://www.unb.ca/biomed/unb_test_of_prosthetics_function.pdf Accessed 14 May 2008

Uswatte G, Miltner WH, Foo B et al (2000) Objective measurement of functional upper-extremity movement using accelerometer recordings transformed with a threshold filter. Stroke 31:662–667

Uswatte G, Foo WL, Olmstead H et al (2005) Ambulatory monitoring of arm movement using accelerometry: an objective measure of upper-extremity rehabilitation in persons with chronic stroke. Arch Phys Med Rehabil 86:1498–1501

van Lunteren A, van Lunteren-Gerritsen GH, Stassen HG, et al (1983) A field evaluation of arm prostheses for unilateral amputees. Prosthet Orthot Int 7:141–151

Vega-Gonzalez A, Granat MH (2005) Continuous monitoring of upper-limb activity in a free-living environment. Arch Phys Med Rehabil 86:541–548

Vlaeyen JW, Van Eek H, Groenman NH et al (1987) Dimensions and components of observed chronic pain behavior. Pain 31:65–75

Weaver SA, Lange LR, Vogts VM (1988) Comparison of myoelectric and conventional prostheses for adolescent amputees. Am J Occup Ther 42:87–91

Welk GJ, Blair SN, Wood K et al (2000) A comparative evaluation of three accelerometry-based physical activity monitors. Med Sci Sports Exerc 32:S489–S497

Wright VF (2006) Measurement of functional outcome with individuals who use upper extremity prosthetic devices: Current and future directions. J Prosth Orthot 18:46–56

Wright TW, Hagen AD, Wood MB (1995) Prosthetic usage in major upper extremity amputations. J Hand Surg [Am] 20:619–622

Wright FV, Hubbard S, Naumann S et al (2003) Evaluation of the validity of the prosthetic upper extremity functional index for children. Arch Phys Med Rehabil 84:518–527

Chapter 5
Adaptation to Amputation and Prosthesis Use

Elisabeth Schaffalitzky, Pamela Gallagher, Deirdre Desmond, and Malcolm MacLachlan

Abstract In this chapter, we focus on psychosocial adaptation to an amputation/absence of a major limb and using a prosthesis. Prosthetic fitting, as a means of addressing cosmesis, functional rehabilitation and quality of life, is the most prevalent form of intervention for people with loss of a body part. However, the ways in which people respond to limb loss and the use of a prosthesis are both complex and individual and can be impacted upon by a variety of personal, clinical, social, physical and environmental factors. We term the study of the psychological, social and behavioural aspects of limb loss and prosthetic use, and of the rehabilitative processes in those conditions that require the use of prosthetic devices *psychoprosthetics*. In this chapter, we develop this concept and explore key issues including adaptation theory, body image, social discomfort and psychosocial factors impacting on adaptation such as coping, social support and culture. This chapter considers the importance of these issues for health service providers across the multidisciplinary team who work with people with limb loss. The integration of an awareness of psychosocial factors in the management of limb loss, together with physical and technical knowledge, is critical to optimising outcomes and enhancing appropriate service provision.

5.1 Introduction

Amputation of a limb is a life-changing event that creates a diversity of different threats and challenges including the physical (e.g., post-operative pain), the financial (e.g., adjusting to potential employment changes), the environmental (e.g., learning to negotiate public transport) and the psychosocial (e.g., emotional consequences, learning to accept a new body image, dealing with perceived or actual

P. Gallagher (✉)
School of Nursing, Dublin City University, Dublin, Ireland
e-mail: pamela.gallagher@dcu.ie

C. Murray (ed.), *Amputation, Prosthesis Use, and Phantom Limb Pain: An Interdiciplinary Perspective*, DOI 10.1007/978-0-387-87462-3_5,

social stigma, a potential loss of independence and changes in social roles). For many people, learning to use a prosthesis is a central consequence of amputation. Indeed, prosthetic fitting, as a means of addressing functional rehabilitation, cosmesis and quality of life, is the most common form of intervention for people with the loss of a body part. Following amputation, there is a period of physical and psychosocial adaptation, and although limb amputation may lead to significant psychosocial dysfunction for some individuals, many others adjust and function well. The ways in which people respond to limb loss and the use of a prosthesis are both complex and individual and can be influenced by a variety of personal, clinical, social, physical and environmental factors. We term the study of the psychological, social, and behavioural aspects of limb loss and prosthetic use, and of the rehabilitative processes in those conditions that require the use of prosthetic devices *Psychoprosthetics* (Gallagher et al. 2008). This chapter provides a brief overview of theory on psychosocial adaptation and issues of affective distress and body image post-amputation. We also consider the role of social support and coping processes in mediating adaptation to amputation and prosthesis use. Finally, we consider the importance of these issues for health service providers across the multidisciplinary team. The integration of an awareness of psychosocial factors in the management of limb loss, together with physical and technical knowledge, is critical to optimising outcomes and enhancing appropriate service provision.

5.2 Adaptation

Psychosocial adaptation to chronic illness and disability can be understood as the process of responding to the psychological, physical, social and environmental changes that occur with the onset and experience of living with a chronic illness or disability (CID) and its associated treatments (Bishop 2005a). People can find themselves with a suddenly or dramatically challenged or even changed sense of self arising from the changes in body image and social roles that can occur (Bishop 2005a). The experiences and meanings that people have built their former self-images upon are no longer available to them as their new reality presents difficulties when trying to maintain their former lives (Charmaz 1983). While adaptation to CID has been an important focus of rehabilitation research for a number of years, Parker et al. (2003) argue that much of the work has been based purely on clinical observation and not empirical findings and that there is little evidence that any theory on adjustment has been effectively transformed into a clinical intervention (Parker et al. 2003). The earliest approaches to psychosocial adjustment to CID tended to be based on a medical or pathological model, which stated that specific types of illness or disability would bring about specific types of reactions or psychological problems. This was basic at best, and completely failed to reflect the complexity and the individuality that exists in the process of adapting to CID. Indeed, using only objectively measured variables based on pathology and disease has been shown to not serve as an important predictor of a patient's overall adaptation (Williamson et al. 1994). Stage theories are based on the concept that there are a predictable number of set stages that an individual has to go through in order to adapt to their illness or disability (e.g. shock, anger, denial etc.). This approach has also been questioned in recent years, especially in terms of progressive illnesses where there can be uncertainty and unpredictability both in terms of the progression of the disease and the individual's reaction to it. Furthermore, it has been argued that the stage models normalise responses such as denial and depression and if these stages are not observed by clinicians, patients may be labelled as "abnormal", leading the model to become a form of social oppression (Parker et al. 2003). Kendall and Buys (1998) also note that stage models are merely descriptive and "provide little information on the factors that contribute to individual differences in the adjustment process, despite the likelihood that these factors will provide the key to maximising the effectiveness of rehabilitation counselling" (p. 17).

Recently, more comprehensive approaches to understanding adaptation have emerged, which reflect the complex nature of adaptation to CID. Livneh (2001) has proposed a model that shows the interactions between antecedent variables (triggering events of CID, e.g., injury leading to amputation, and contextual variables, e.g., psychosocial status) and process variables (contextual influences, e.g., personality traits and the influence they exert on adaptation, and experienced reactions, i.e., short- and long-term psychosocial reactions to CID) and illustrates how these interactions will influence outcomes (most notably Quality of Life). Bishop has put forward a model called "Disability Centrality" (Bishop 2005a, b) which is based on the fact that quality of life is determined by different domains having different levels of importance for every individual, and that disruption of the more important domains has an effect on the quality of life. Citing the work of Maslow and Rogers, Bishop argues that as we strive for higher quality of life, we need to make adaptive changes in either domain importance or domain control. This model is similar to the work of Charmaz (1983), who uses former identities rather than domains, as the area that needs to be changed to adapt to the differences arising from CID. For example, a person may place less importance on their former identity as an employed person as they are no longer able to work. Despite the ongoing debates about the adaptation process, there are two points of general consensus that have emerged: (a) adaptation to CID involves a multidimensional response, i.e., CID effects a number of different domains, thus adaptation will involve a number of different domains, (b) adaptation is a subjective process, i.e., the individual's personal, subjective examination of his or her circumstances will be the most important factor in leading to an adaptation response (Bishop 2005a). Both of these highlight the need to not only study a number of different psychosocial processes in relation to adaptation to amputation but to include the perspective of the person adapting. In keeping with this, Rybarczyk et al. (2004) have noted that the physical aspects of a disability are much less important to the adaptation process than are psychological, developmental and social environmental factors, as well as resources of the individual who acquires the disability.

With regard to adapting to the prosthesis, despite the best efforts of the rehabilitation team, there are a number of people who will persistently return with problems and who may eventually abandon the prosthesis. In a study of 396 individuals with lower limb amputations in Canada (Gauthier-Gagnon et al. 1998), it was reported that 28.5% of non-users rejected their prosthesis because it no longer fit, yet refused to return it for repairs, or adjustments, even when the prosthetist was nearby and appointments were readily available to the patient. Prosthesis abandonment is not only related to the fit of the prosthesis, but potentially to other factors that could be psychological in nature. Marcia Scherer has created a model for Matching Person with Technology (MPT) (Scherer 2000). MPT takes into account not only the salient characteristics of the assistive technology itself, but also the characteristics of the environment and the situations in which the technology is to be used, and the relevant features of the individual's personality, temperament and preferences that may have an effect on the use of the technology. She argues that an individual may be an optimal user according to one or two of the factors, but may be a reluctant user on the other factor. For example, they may have the optimal personality and technology factors, but be reluctant to use their technology because of the lack of support in their environment from family and friends. As such, the environment for use will need to be modified so the individual can gain optimal satisfaction and functional gain from the device. Assistive device use is also seen as dynamic and interactive, changes in one set of factors impact on the other factors. For example, if an individual feels they have the best technology available and feel no discomfort or pain using it, they may become proud of using the device and improve their self-confidence, maybe in turn broadening their involvement in the community.

In both the research literature and in practice, the terms adapting to an amputation and adapting to a prosthesis are often used interchangeably. Although closely linked, and for many co-occurring, it is important to note that they are not synonymous. Adaptation to amputation does not necessitate prosthesis use. Many individuals accept their amputation as part of their life and adapt well to their new reality, yet choose not to use a prosthesis. Indeed, Heinemann and Pape (2002) state that device user rates are greater when users participate in device selection, the device is easy to use and aesthetically pleasing, the time required for activity completion is perceived as being reasonable, and when the person has also achieved a sufficient level of adaptation to the disability. Given the short time frame post-amputation in which individuals are typically encouraged to start using their prostheses, it is likely that adaptation to amputation concurrently involves the acceptance of the prosthesis into the life of the user. Thus, adapting to a prosthesis involves an interaction between adaptation to amputation and the individual meanings that a person ascribes to the prosthesis, their self, and the society that they live in.

5.2.1 Emotional Well-being

Changes in self-concept following amputation may challenge an individual's ability to maintain emotional well-being and may stimulate maladaptive reactions leading to poor psychosocial adjustment, which may further affect rehabilitation potential and quality of life. Depression is a common experience after limb loss; symptoms of anxiety are likely to be increased in the period immediately after and up to 1 year post-amputation, typically returning to population levels thereafter (Horgan and MacLachlan 2004). Few studies have assessed Post-Traumatic Stress Disorder (PTSD) following amputation. Recently, Phelps et al. (2008) studied people at 6 and 12 months post-amputation for symptoms of depression using the Patient Health Questionnaire-9 (Spitzer et al. 1999) and PTSD using the PTSD Checklist (PCL) (Weathers et al. 1993). At 6 months, 10.8% of the sample of 83 adults reported symptoms consistent with a diagnosis of major depression and a further 4.8% reported minor depression. At 12 months, 12.8% reported symptoms consistent with a diagnosis of major depression and 64% minor depression. In terms of PTSD, at 6 months, 22.9% reported symptoms consistent with a diagnosis of PTSD and at 12 months, 26% reported symptoms consistent with a diagnosis of PTSD.

5.2.2 Body Image, Stigma and Social Discomfort

The person who has experienced an amputation must adjust to a number of different body images including the "complete" or familiar body prior to the limb loss, the traumatised body, the healing body and the extended body, that is, a body supplemented with prosthetic devices and, if necessary, other types of assistive technology, or indeed a body that has been extended beyond its existing physical boundaries as a result of phantom sensations and/or phantom limb pain (i.e., sensations and/or pain, respectively in the part of the body that has been amputated) (Gallagher et al. 2007). According to Rybarczyk et al. (2000) the person has to adapt to an image of themselves without the amputated limb while reconciling three images of their body: before the limb loss, without a prosthesis, and with a prosthesis. For people with an amputation, there are visible differences in their physical appearance to themselves. The visibility of physical difference to others can depend on the type and location of amputation, the type of activity undertaken and clothing choices. After an amputation, individuals may undertake activities in different ways or may move differently. Such differences can lead to self-consciousness and to feelings of stigmatisation by others or the self. Taleporos and McCabe (2002) argue that being stigmatised by others may lead to feelings of being discounted socially, financially, and intellectually purely on the basis of physical appearance. In this way, the disability can become the over-riding identity obscuring all other personal characteristics, skills and abilities. The individuals themselves may also take this view as the physical form affects self-perceived capability and acceptability to others (Breakey 1997). This may be further affected by the use of a mobility aid, as in general, mobility aids are associated with aging and disability (Aminzadeh and Edwards 1998). Cultural norms can also influence the incorporation of a disability into one's self-concept and in turn affect acceptance of a disability (Jonsson et al. 1999). These will often dictate social roles, activities in which persons are expected to function, and consequently the readiness to accommodate disability within the experience of self (Pape et al. 2002).

Feeling stigmatised may lead individuals to avoid certain social situations such as those revealing the body (Donovan-Hall et al. 2002; Sjodahl et al. 2004) and lead to feelings of social discomfort (Rybarczyk et al. 1992). Rybarczyk et al. (1992) asked 89 people with amputations whether they were bothered by public enquiries about their amputation or prosthesis, and if they avoided being in public because of their amputation or prosthesis. They found that a high level of social discomfort was a significant predictor of depression, even after the effects of age, gender, social support, time since amputation, reason for amputation and perceived health were controlled. Furthermore, Gallagher and MacLachlan (2001) reported that focus group participants recounted awkward situations when they told people about having a prosthetic limb, their concern about the impression they made on others and the wish to appear "normal". Indeed, a relationship between high public self-consciousness and greater restriction of normal activities such as self-care and visiting friends has been found (Williamson 1995) indicating the importance of body image in social functioning. Rybarczyk et al. (1997) theorise that when certain activities that are essential to an individual's identity and self-worth are threatened, such as their employment status or recreation activities (social functioning), the individual will feel demoralised and may become depressed. This is in keeping with the previously discussed work of Charmaz (1995) and Bishop (2005a, b), that is, an individual may need to change how important CID-affected domains in life are to them, or place less importance on the CID-affected identities they used to inhabit if they wish to adapt and move on. Conversely, individuals may have less difficulty adjusting to their amputation if they have fewer activities that are restricted from their life pre-amputation, e.g., if they had a sedentary lifestyle pre-amputation, they may see no need for a prosthetic to aid ambulation.

Apart from the stigmatisations that can arise from disability, other problems relate to body image. Certain body parts carry conscious and unconscious symbolic meaning for an individual (Breakey 1997) and bodily appearance affects both social identifications and self-definitions (Charmaz 1995). Consequently, there appears to be a relationship between how a person perceives his/her body image and psychological well-being. Rybarczyk et al. (1995) conducted a study with 112 people with lower limb amputations and found that body image and perceived social stigma were significant and independent predictors of depression after controlling for factors found to be linked to adjustment in previous studies (such as time since amputation, site of amputation and cause of amputation). Perceived social stigma was the best predictor of depression. Body image was also found to be an independent predictor of quality of life and an individual's prosthetists' rating of his or her psychological adjustment.

Gender differences have emerged with regard to body image and prosthesis satisfaction. On the basis of 44 responses to an internet survey incorporating the

Trinity Amputation and Prosthesis Experience Scales (TAPES) (Gallagher and MacLachlan 2000a), the Amputee Body Image Scale (ABIS) (Breakey 1997) and the McGill pain questionnaire (MPQ) (Melzack 1975), Murray and Fox (2002) found that higher levels of functional satisfaction with their prosthesis were correlated with lower levels of body image disturbance in men. However, in women, higher levels of functional satisfaction, aesthetic satisfaction, and weight satisfaction, were associated with lower levels of body image disturbance. Taking the sample as a whole, higher levels of overall satisfaction and functional satisfaction with a prosthesis and lower levels of body image disturbance, were correlated with higher levels of hourly prosthesis use per day. This can be interpreted in two ways: using the prosthesis more results in a better body image or a better body image results in more prosthesis use. Analyses based on gender revealed that only higher functional satisfaction with the prosthesis was correlated with daily hours of prosthetic use in males, while greater prosthetic use in females was correlated with higher functional, aesthetic and weight satisfaction with the prosthesis. For male participants, functionality was important, perhaps relating to traditional social roles. For females, it appears that the aesthetics are important perhaps through helping to sustain a sense of femininity. This is similar to findings that young people and women, but not older men, are more likely to feel their choice of apparel is affected by the use of a prosthesis (Nicholas et al. 1993).

5.2.3 *Summary*

Limb loss has a transformative role in self-concept, necessitating a renegotiation of the self in the social world. The way in which a person with an amputation experiences the self and their construction of meaning from experience, influences their attitudes towards prosthetic devices and subsequent prosthetic usage. Difficulties in integrating and adapting prosthetic technology into an individual's life may result from difficulties in integrating post-amputation changes into self-concept (MacLachlan and Gallagher 2004).

5.3 Psychosocial Factors Impacting on Adaptation

Models describing individual differences in psychological adjustment to CID implicate a complex interplay among risk factors, resource or resistance factors, intrapersonal factors and social-ecological factors. Here, we describe the role of coping, social support, and cultural factors in adjustment to amputation and prosthesis use.

5.3.1 *Coping*

Coping strategies are used in situations in which there is a perceived discrepancy between stressful demands and available resources for meeting these demands (Zeidner and Endler 1996). Within the coping literature, there is a broad distinction between "problem-focused coping" strategies, such as confronting, planned problem solving and seeking social support, and "emotion-focused coping" strategies such as self regulation of emotions, distancing, positive reappraisal, accepting responsibility and avoidance.

Coping with limb loss involves multiple demands, both physical and psychological. Research that specifically evaluates the role of coping strategies in amputation adjustment is consistent with the general coping literature, suggesting that active and task orientated coping strategies, such as problem solving, are conducive to positive psychosocial adjustment, while emotion-focused coping and cognitive disengagement are positively associated with anxiety, depression, and externalised hostility and negatively associated with acceptance of disability (Livneh et al. 1999; Desmond and MacLachlan 2006). The specific coping strategy of catastrophising is also associated with higher levels of pain severity and poor adjustment to chronic pain and was the single most important predictor of current pain, pain interference, depression and future pain interference (Jensen et al. 2002) in a study of adjustment to phantom limb pain.

Dunn (1996) investigated the influence of three different coping modes, namely finding positive meaning, dispositional optimism and perceiving control over disability, on depression and self-esteem in adjustment to amputation. Finding positive meaning in one's amputation was associated with lower levels of depressive symptomatology, and perceiving greater control over one's impairment and dispositional optimism were associated with lower levels of depressive symptomatology and higher levels of self esteem after an amputation. Finding positive meaning after amputation has also been found to be associated with more favourable health and physical capabilities, higher adjustment to limitation and lower athletic activity restriction (as measured by the TAPES) (Gallagher and MacLachlan 2000b). In both studies, finding positive meaning was described as taking a variety of different forms, such as re-evaluating the event as positive, redefining the amputation in one's life, finding side benefits such as meeting new people, imagining worse situations or making favourable social comparisons (Dunn 1996, Gallagher and MacLachlan 2000b). Phelps et al. (2008) reported that being positive about the amputation (positive cognitive processing) was predictive of post-traumatic growth, i.e., a shift in how individuals view themselves, their priorities and interactions with others.

Many of the above strategies are consistent with Sjodahl et al.'s (2004) description of selective evaluation. This is explained as a cognitive mechanism used to support the person by appraising themselves and/or their situation in comparison to chosen norms. There are five mechanisms of selective evaluation:

1. to make comparison with more unfortunate persons (downward comparisons)
2. to selectively focus on dimensions to make your own situation more favourable

3. to create a hypothetically worse situation (what might have happened)
4. to invent benefits from the experience
5. to create norms as a standard which makes your own adjustments seem exceptional (Taylor et al. 1983).

Selective evaluation is rooted in Festinger's (1954) social comparison theory which states that people compare themselves to others either by making upward comparisons to people better off, or downward comparisons to people who are worse off than themselves. These comparisons affect self-esteem, mental health and other aspects of behaviour, especially when considered in health and health care (Skevington 2004). Comparisons can be made between people who are within the same group, e.g., people with amputations, and also between people in different groups, e.g., between a person with an amputation and a person in a burn unit. Making downward social comparisons can aid the adjustment to a range of negative events (Taylor and Lobel 1989). However, it has been recognised that social comparisons are a short-term rather than long-tem coping response as they only serve to improve mood and boost self-evaluations and thus do not provide information about successful adjustment (Dunn 1996). Sjodahl et al. (2004) found that people with traumatic or tumour-related lower limb amputation used downward comparisons with others more ill or more unfortunate than themselves to strengthen their self-confidence. On discharge, however, comparisons shifted and centred on the contrast between life pre-amputation and the new reality as a person with an amputation. Coping strategies that are adaptive at one point in time may become less frequently used or may even have different effects if adopted at different times (Oaksford et al. 2005). For example, a problem-solving strategy that causes the person to engage in exercise on a tender stump may result in the person experiencing other types of pain (Gallagher and MacLachlan 1999).

5.3.2 Social Support

The quantity and quality of social relationships affect health and well-being. For example, people with larger social networks and stronger social bonds within their networks have better physical and mental health, fewer illnesses, quicker recovery from physical and psychological problems, and less depression (Saranson et al. 1990). Social support may take many forms, such as easing the stressor with companionship, offering ideas for coping or even just giving reassurance that you are cared about and valued as a person and that everything will be all right (Saranson et al. 1997). The mechanisms whereby social support enhances well-being have been characterised in terms of main and buffering effects. By mediating the relationship between stressful life events and psychological distress, social support can influence the individual's appraisal of the potential stressor, i.e., it acts as a buffer. Alternatively, social support can have a "direct effect", the main effect hypothesis, in that it will have an effect on well-being regardless of the stressor involved and that the absence of social support can in and of itself act as a stressor (Schwarzer et al. 2004).

Social support is usually measured in studies as perceived social support, that is, how the individual sees the support network available to them. It is suggested that perceived support will have a main effect on psychological well-being whereas received support will have a buffering effect (Cohen and Willis 1985). Rook (1990) maintains that health and well-being are not merely the result of actual support provision but are the outcomes of participation in a meaningful social context. Essentially, being embedded in a positive social world that involves receiving and giving support and companionship might be more influential than just receiving help.

Within the amputation and prosthetics field, social support is increasingly recognised as a predictor of better outcomes. For instance, Darnall et al. (2005) identified that a person with an amputation who was divorced or separated had an increased risk of depressive symptoms compared with a person who was married or partnered. This was consistent with an earlier study by Nielson (1991) who reported significantly higher levels of life satisfaction in people with an amputation who were married than those who were unmarried. Perceived social support has been linked with quality of life (Rybarczyk et al. 1995), a decrease in levels of depression and future improvement in phantom limb pain interference (Jensen et al. 2002).

Social support can also be measured by looking at a person's social integration, i.e., the extent to which an individual participates in a broad range of social relationships (this includes behavioural (actively engaging in activities with others) and cognitive (sense of place within the community components) (Williams et al. 2004). In a sample of people with a new lower limb amputation, Williams et al. (2004) reported that while overall social integration did not change significantly over the first year post-amputation and was not related to gender, partner/living status or amputation aetiology, at 24 months post-amputation, persons who were married or living with a romantic partner reported greater social integration than those unmarried or living alone. Age was also found to be related to social integration, with levels of social integration decreasing as age increased. Considering the impact of social integration and perceived social support on outcomes, social integration was significantly related to occupational status one month after amputation but was not as important as perceived social support in predicting outcomes such as quality of life, depression, pain interference and mobility. Therefore, Williams and colleagues concluded that the quality of relationships, rather than the quantity of social network interactions were better determinants of how an individual will cope with the loss of a limb.

Although social support is predominantly a positive factor, if social support is solicitous, that is overly attentive or overly concerned, or not of a significant quality, it can result in negative outcomes. Solicitous spouse responses were associated with increased levels of depression and phantom limb pain at one month post-amputation (Jensen et al. 2002). A person may cultivate feelings of worthlessness through over reliance on help from others, or may experience distress as a result of receiving unwanted assistance. Thus, social support may be unintentionally de-motivating and may lead to learned helplessness.

5.4 Cultural Factors

There is very little work on broader sociocultural or contextual aspects of prosthetic use even though it is well established that cultural factors can affect the cause, experience, expression and consequence of disease and disability more generally (MacLachlan 2004, 2006). Given the "burden of disease" associated with disability, and its patterning according to socioeconomic factors, particularly in low-income countries (MacLachlan and Swartz 2009), this is an area that needs much greater research. Murray has argued for greater recognition of the gendering of prosthetic use, where men may, for instance, put greater emphasis on functionality and women put a greater emphasis on aesthetics (Murray 2008). He cites the case of one woman who was angry because she was prescribed a man's foot (the only available) and another where a women felt that wearing a prosthetic hook was less socially acceptable for women than it was for men. Similarly, Murray notes the case of a black woman in the UK who was offered a pink, rather than a black, prosthetic foot, and the consequent distress this caused her.

In addition to the need to understand the consequences of different cultural readings of amputation and prosthetic use, there is also a need to consider how contextual factors, especially in very resource poor areas, may affect prosthetic use (Eide and Øderud 2009). Many wheelchairs are, for instance, rendered useless in rural areas with very poor roads and pathways. Similarly, the lack of technical support facilities for prosthetic users can limit the usefulness of such devices; in may cases using a crutch can be a more practical, low cost and durable form of assistive "technology". Ironically, the visibility of a crutch can be of economic benefit because it can contribute to the justification for begging, while a prosthesis may be seen as a sign of "having been taken care of" rather than in "want".

While we tend to think of the effects of culture between ethnic groups, organisational culture is also important. For instance, in many health services, persons with amputations are referred to as "amputees". Although the origins of this terminology is readily understandable within the clinical context, it does nonetheless, literally, refer to people by what they have not got, rather than by who they are or what they have got. The terms invalid (in-valid) or handicap (cap-in-hand, i.e., begging) are social constructions of people which we now recognize as being derogatory. The United Nations Declaration of the Rights of Persons with Disability (UNDRPD) stresses the rights of people as persons first, and secondly as people with disabilities. Admittedly, some linguistic constructions seem more awkward and less "natural" than others, but this also reflects a socialisation which constructs people primarily by their differences, rather than primarily as people (with secondary associated characteristics). Health service cultures should be reflexive and consider how best to refer to those they are seeking to help. We would suggest cultivating an environment where being a "person with an amputation" is a more familiar linguistic construction, than the undeniably truncated, "amputee" construction.

5.5 Importance for Health Service Providers

Greater understanding of the psychological and social realities of limb loss and prosthetic use can contribute to a holistic rehabilitation and limb-fitting experience. An awareness of psychosocial issues in amputation and rehabilitation is critical to optimising patient outcomes and enhancing appropriate service provision. Wegener et al. (2008) propose that attention to psychosocial variables is a shared responsibility of all rehabilitation team members and invoke the PLISSIT model, as a model for team involvement in psychological care (for a full discussion of the model in amputation rehabilitation see Wegnner et al. 2008). The model is not a diagnostic tool but a way of gathering information to facilitate provision of appropriate intervention (Wallace 2003). The PLISSIT acronym signifies four levels of intervention that are based on the skills and comfort of providers and the needs of patients: Permission (P), Limited Information (LI), Specific Suggestions (SS) and Intensive Therapy (IT). Permission giving involves allowing patients to have psychosocial concerns and proactively creating opportunities for discussion of psychosocial issues. Wegener et al. note that in many cases creating an opportunity to discuss psychosocial concerns is sufficient and further intervention is often not necessary. However, for some additional steps are required. Limited information refers to the provision of general information and strategies regarding psychosocial issues, whereas specific suggestions involve focused intervention to address a particular problem. The intensive therapy aspect of the model relates to formal psychotherapeutic intervention. Across this continuum of care practitioners must recognize their own strengths and limitations and acknowledge the limits of their own expertise, providing appropriate referral to those more able to address patients' individual needs where necessary.

The psychosocial aspects of adaptation to amputation and prosthetic use are central to constructing and implementing a rehabilitation plan for persons with amputations. However, as well as being critical at this instrumental level, it also has a critical role in promoting a positive embodied experience of prosthetic use (MacLachlan 2004; MacLachlan and Gallagher 2004; Murray 2008). What, we may ask, is embodied in the use of a prosthetic device? For some, it may represent their inability to perform certain activities; it may be a focus for perceived stigma associated with their physical condition, and it may emphasis their lack of completeness. Yet for others, a prosthetic device may represent their enablement; their ability to harness technology, to fully participate in society and to be more than they could be without it. How people "read" their prosthetic device is potentially one of the most powerful psychosocial factors in their rehabilitation. This is a factor that all health professionals can influence, by taking into account the explicit factors described in this chapter, and also their own implicit psychology, in their inter-action with prosthetic users.

5.6 Conclusion

Amputation confronts individuals with an evolving spectrum of challenges. The ways in which people respond to limb loss and prosthetic use are both complex and individual and are characterised in part by time, physical factors, context (including developmental stage, gender and cultural heritage), resources, and intrapersonal factors. Emphasising psychosocial factors across the continuum of care can serve to support positive adaptation and to improve outcomes and service delivery.

References

Aminzadeh RN, Edwards R (1998) Exploring seniors' views on the use of assistive devices in fall prevention. Public Health Nurs 15:297–305

Bishop M (2005a) Quality of life and psychosocial adaptation to chronic illness and acquired disability: a conceptual and theoretical synthesis. J Rehabil 71:5–13

Bishop M (2005b) Quality of life and psychosocial adaptation to chronic illness and disability: preliminary analysis of a conceptual and theoretical synthesis. Rehabil Couns Bull 48:219–231

Breakey JW (1997) Body image: the lower-limb amputee. J Prosthet Orthot 9:58–66

Charmaz K (1983) Loss of self: a fundamental form of suffering in the chronically ill. Sociol Health Illn 5:168–197

Charmaz K (1995) The body, identity and self: adapting to impairment. Sociol Q 36:657–680

Cohen S, Willis TA (1985) Stress, social support, and the buffering hypothesis. Psychol Bull 98:310–357

Darnall BD, Ephraim PL, Wegener ST, Dillingham TR, Pezzin LE, Rossbach P, Mackenzie EJ (2005) Depressive symptoms and mental health service utilisation among persons with limb loss: results of a national survey. Arch Phys Med Rehabil 86:650–658

Desmond D, MacLachlan M (2006) Coping strategies as predictors of psychosocial adaptation in a sample of elderly veterans with acquired lower limb amputations. Soc Sci Med 62:208–216

Donovan-Hall MK, Yardley L, Watts RJ (2002) Engagement in activities revealing the body and psychosocial adjustment in adults with a trans-tibial prosthesis. Prosthet Orthot Int 26:15–22

Dunn DS (1996) Well-being following amputation: salutary effects of positive meaning, optimism, and control. Rehabil Psychol 41:285–302

Eide AH, Øderud T (2009) Assistive technology in low income countries. In: MacLachlan M, Swartz L (eds) Disability and international development: towards inclusive global health. Springer, New York

Festinger L (1954) A theory of social comparison processes. Hum Relat 7:117–140

Gallagher P, Desmond D, MacLachlan M (2008) Psychoprosthetics: an Introduction. In: Gallagher P, Desmond D, MacLachlan M (eds) Psychoprosthetics. Springer, London

Gallagher P, MacLachlan M (1999) Psychological adjustment and coping in adults with prosthetic limbs. Behav Med 25:117–124

Gallagher P, MacLachlan M (2000a) Development and psychometric evaluation of the Trinity Amputation and Prosthesis Scales (TAPES). Rehabil Psychol 45:130–154

Gallagher P, MacLachlan M (2000b) Positive meaning in amputation and thoughts about the amputated limb. Prosthet Orthot Int 24:196–204

Gallagher P, MacLachlan M (2001) Adjustment to an artificial limb: a qualitative perspective. J Health Psychol 6:85–100

Gallagher P, Horgan O, Franchignoni F, Giordano A, Maclachlan M (2007) Body Image in People with Lower-Limb Amputation: A Rasch Analysis of the Amputee Body Image Scale. Am J Phys Med 86:205–215

Gauthier-Gagnon C, Grise MC, Potvin D (1998) Predisposing factors related to prosthetic use by people with a transtibial and transfemoral amputation. J Prosthet Orthot 10:99–109

Heinemann AW, Pape TL-B (2002) Coping and adjustment. In: Scherer MJ (ed) Assistive technology. Matching device and consumer for successful rehabilitation. American Psychological Association, Washington, DC

Horgan O, MacLachlan M (2004) Psychological adjustment to lower-limb amputation: a review. Disabil Rehabil 26:837–850

Jensen MP, Ehde DM, Hoffman AJ, Patterson DR, Czerniecki JM, Robinson LR (2002) Cognitions, coping and social environment predict adjustment to phantom limb pain. Pain 95:133–142

Jonsson A, Moller A, Grimby G (1999) Managing occupations in everyday life to achieve adaptation. Am J Occup Ther 53:353–362

Kendall E, Buys N (1998) An integrated model for psychosocial adjustment following acquired disability. J Rehabil 64:16–20

Livneh H (2001) Psychosocial adaptation to chronic illness and disability: a conceptual framework. Rehabil Couns Bull 44:151–160

Livneh H, Aantnak RF, Gerhardt J (1999) Psychosocial adaptation to amputation: the role of sociodemographic variables, disability related factors and coping strategies. Int J Rehabil Res 22:21–31

MacLachlan M, Gallagher P (2004) Imagining the body. In: Gallagher P, MacLachlan M (eds) Enabling technologies: body image and body function. Edinburgh, Churchill-Livingstone, pp 3–20

MacLachlan M (2004) Embodiment: clinical, critical and cultural perspectives on health and illness. Open University Press, Milton Keynes

MacLachlan M (2006) Culture and health: a critical perspective towards global health. Wiley, Chichester

MacLachlan M, Swartz L (eds) (2009) Disability and international development: towards inclusive global health. Springer, New York

Melzack R (1975) The McGill pain questionnaire: major properties and scoring methods. Pain 1:255–299

Murray C, Fox J (2002) Body image and prosthesis satisfaction in the lower limb amputee. Disabil Rehabil 24:925–931

Murray CD (2008) Embodiment and prosthetics. In: Gallagher P, Desmond D, MacLachlan M (eds) Psychoprosthetics. Springer, London

Nicholas JJ, Robinson LR, Schulz R, Blair C, Aliota R, Hairston G (1993) Problems experienced and perceived by prosthetic patients. J Prosthet Orthot 5:16–19

Nielson CC (1991) A survey of amputees: functional level and life satisfaction, information needs and the prosthetist's role. J Prosthet Orthot 3:125–129

Oaksford K, Frude N, Cuddihy R (2005) Positive coping and stress-related psychological growth following lower-limb amputation. Rehabil Psychol 50:266–277

Pape TL-B, Kim J, Weiner B (2002) The shaping of individual meanings assigned to assistive technology: a review of personal factors. Disabil Rehabil 24:5–20

Parker RM, Schaller J, Hansmann S (2003) Catastrophe, chaos and complexity models and psychosocial adjustment to disability. Rehabil Couns Bull 46:234–251

Phelps LF, Williams RM, Raichle KA, Turner AP, Ehde DM (2008) The importance of cognitive processing to adjustment in the 1st year following amputation. Rehabil Psychol 53:28–38

Rook KS (1990) Social relationships as a source of companionship: implications for older adults' psychological well being. In: Saranson BR, Saranson IG, Pierce GR (eds) Social support: an international view. Wiley, New York

Rybarczyk B, Edwards R, Behal J (2004) Diversity in adjustment to a leg amputation: case illustrations of common themes. Disabil Rehabil 26:944–953

Rybarczyk B, Nicholas JJ, Nyenhuis D (1997) Coping with a leg amputation: integration research and clinical practice. Rehabil Psychol 42:241–256
Rybarczyk B, Nyenhuis D, Knussen C, Nicholas JJ, Cash SM, Kaiser J (1995) Body image, perceived social stigma, and the prediction of psychosocial adjustment to leg amputation. Rehabil Psychol 49:95–110
Rybarczyk B, Nyenhuis D, Nicholas JJ, Schulz R, Aliota R, Blair C (1992) Social discomfort and depression in a sample of adults with leg amputations. Arch Phys Med Rehabil 73:1169–1173
Rybarczyk B, Szymanski L, Nicholas JJ (2000) Psychological adjustment to a limb amputation. In: Frank R, Elliott T (eds) Handbook of rehabilitation psychology. American Psychological Association, Washington, DC
Saranson B, Saranson I, Pierce G (1990) Social support: an international review. Wiley, New York
Saranson B, Saranson IG, Gurung RAR (1997) Close personal relationships and health outcomes: a key to the role of social support. In: Duck S (ed) Handbook of personal relationships, 2nd edn. Wiley, Chichester, UK
Scherer MJ (2000) Living in the state of stuck: how assistive technology impacts the lives of people with disabilities. Brookline Books, Cambridge, MA
Schwarzer R, Knoll N, Rieckmann N (2004) Social support. In: Kapttein A, Weinman J (eds) Health psychology. BPS Blackwell, Oxford
Sjodahl C, Gard G, Jarnlo G-B (2004) Coping after trans-femoral amputation due to trauma or tumour – a phenomenological approach. Disabil Rehabil 26:851–861
Skevington SM (2004) Pain and symptom perception. In: Kaptein A, Weinman J (eds) Health psychology. BPS Blackwell, Oxford
Spitzer RL, Kroenke K, Williams JBW (1999) Validation and utility of a self-report version of the PRIME-MD. J Am Med Assoc 282:1749–1756
Taleporos G, McCabe MP (2002) Body image and physical disability – personal perspectives. Soc Sci Med 54:971–980
Taylor SE, Lobel M (1989) Social comparison activity under threat: downward evaluation and upward contacts. Psychol Rev 96:569–575
Taylor SE, Wood JV, Lichtman RR (1983) It could be worse: selective evaluation as a response to victimization. J Soc Issues 39:19–40
Wallace M (2003) Try this. Best practices in nursing care to older adults: sexuality. Derm Nurs 15:570–571
Weathers FW, Litz BT, Herman DS, Huska JA, Keane TM (1993) The PTSD checklist: reliability, validity, and diagnostic utility. Annual meeting of the international society for traumatic stress studies, San Antonio, Texas
Wegnner SW, Hofkamp SE, Ehde DM (2008) Interventions for psychological issues in amputation: a team approach. In: Gallagher P, Desmond D, MacLachlan M (eds) Psychoprosthetics. Springer, London
Williams RM, Ehde DM, Smith DG, Czernieski JM, Hoffman AJ, Robinson LR (2004) A two-year longitudinal study of social support following amputation. Disabil Rehabil 26:962–874
Williamson GM (1995) Restrictions of normal activities among older adult amputees: the role of public self-consciousness. J Clin Geropsychol 1:229–242
Williamson GM, Schulz R, Bridges MW, Behan AM (1994) Social and psychological factors in adjustment to limb amputation. J Soc Behav Pers 9:249–268
Zeidner M, Endler N (1996) Handbook of coping: theory, research, applications. Wiley, New York

Chapter 6
Understanding Adjustment and Coping to Limb Loss and Absence through Phenomenologies of Prosthesis Use

Craig Murray

Abstract "Adjustment" and "coping" are two interrelated psychologically based concepts which have been applied and explored extensively in research on chronic illness and disability. These areas are often explored using structured, quantitative research methods, where coping and adapting are seen as final adaptive steps or stages made in response to ill health or disability. These concepts and methodological frameworks have similarly been used to explore amputation, congenital limb deficiency or absence and prosthesis use. However, more recently researchers have begun to use phenomenologically based qualitative methods to explore the meanings and experience of illness and disability from the vantage point of those concerned, so that what it is to cope or adapt, and how this is negotiated, is informed by the perspectives of those having the relevant experience rather than through the application of priori theoretical frameworks. Within this chapter, I summarise the findings of a large-scale project, which aimed to explore the meanings and experience of prosthesis use for both people with acquired amputation and congenital limb absence or deformity. The key theme domains to be identified in this work are the embodied experience, personal and social meanings of prosthesis use. This work highlights the subtle and complex ways in which such persons manage, negotiate and experience their identity in everyday life, and therefore how they adapt to and cope with their changing circumstances. The outcomes of this work have a number of implications for health professionals working with this client group which are discussed.

6.1 Introduction

There is now a large body of quantitative literature on issues such as "adjustment" (see Horgan and MacLachlan 2004) and "coping" (e.g. Desmond 2007) to amputation and prosthesis use. This literature tends to conceptualise these topics as psychological

C.D. Murray
School of Health and Medicine, Lancaster University, Lancaster, UK
e-mail: c.murray@lancaster.ac.uk

C. Murray (ed.), *Amputation, Prosthesis Use, and Phantom Limb Pain: An Interdisciplinary Perspective*, DOI 10.1007/978-0-387-87462-3_6,

states to be successfully achieved, so that someone who adjusts and copes with limb loss and prosthesis use is someone who has made adaptive psychological changes to their circumstances. An example of this way of conceptualising adapting to or coping with amputation is evident in a recent paper by Schulz (2009: 74):

> "It is important for the amputees to go through the different stages of mourning: The first stage is the rejection of the situation. Repression and denial of the loss protects the patient from emotional overstrain. Confrontation is the next step: emotionally as well as mentally. "How could it happen?", (understanding the reasons why ...) "What will my future be like?", "How will I cope?" (ability of coping) "Why did it happen to me?" (sense) The last stage of coping with the amputation is to accept and deal with the new situation and to build up new self-confidence. A successful process of coping leads to a new identity."

Such structured quantitative approaches to adapting to or coping with amputation tend to view these as final steps or stages in a process of psychological change. What such approaches often overlook is exactly what it is to "cope" or "adjust" for those concerned, and how these might be psychologically and pragmatically achieved. As Horgan and MacLachlan (2004) acknowledge, previous work in these areas have not paid a great deal of attention to more immediate reactions to amputation, adjustment during and shortly after the rehabilitation period, or how a sense of self and identity changes and develops post-amputation. These authors recommended that more longitudinal and qualitative research was needed to appropriately address these research areas.

Indeed, in response to such quantitative approaches to adjustment and coping in health and disability research, some researchers have sought alternative research methods to enable the identification, from the viewpoints of those concerned, of what the meanings of ill health and disability are, and not only *how* such people cope or adjust, but *what it is* to cope and adjust for them. However, in contrast to the relatively large quantitative literature on coping and adjustment, there is only a small literature available from a qualitative perspective. The nature of phenomenologically oriented qualitative work, namely those branches of qualitative inquiry concerned with the exploration of experiences and meanings within the contexts in which they arise, means that it is well suited to elaborating the experience of amputation and prosthesis use from the vantage point of prosthesis users. The importance of such an endeavour is supported by the work of Dunn (1996), who found the very process of "finding meaning" following amputation to be linked to lower levels of depressive symptomatology. Therefore, understanding the experiences of those with recent amputations beginning to use a prosthesis, as well as established prosthesis users (as well as those somewhere in between), may inform and facilitate the work of a variety of health professionals involved in the rehabilitative process.

Existing qualitative literature has addressed the personal meanings of choosing *not* to use prosthetic limbs. The key work here is that of Gelya Frank, who has elaborated how people with congenital limb deficiencies may challenge the stigmatisation of their condition (Frank 1986), and the way in which "rejection" of prosthetic limbs can constitute a positive decision (Frank 1988). Similar first-person accounts of prosthesis *use* are rare. However, recently a small body of qualitative literature looking at amputation and prosthesis use has emerged. For example,

Gallagher and MacLachlan (2001) took a qualitative approach to identify factors considered important by persons with limb loss in their adjustment to amputation and prosthesis use. Using a focus group methodology, they explored the experiences of younger lower-limb amputees and used thematic analysis to identify issues of importance in the adjustment process. In their discussion of their data, Gallagher and MacLachlan argued that adjustment to limb loss and prosthesis use is complex and long term.

Oaksford et al. (2005) used the qualitative method of grounded theory to explore positive coping and stress-related psychological growth following lower limb amputation. They asked participants to explicitly reflect upon their personal coping style and to describe the strategies they used when coping with their amputation. They concluded that coping strategies evolve to reflect post amputation changes in psychological demands. Similarly, Saradjian et al. (2008) explored the experience of males using an upper limb prosthesis following amputation, and described themes of psychosocial and functional adjustment to minimize a sense of difference in appearance and ability. Adjustment was facilitated by the personal meanings of participants' prostheses and their positive coping styles.

The above work has been useful in broadening and deepening an understanding of how coping or adjustment is actually experienced and achieved, and indicates a more complex way of conceptualising just what these terms refer to and how rather than being end-state achievements, "adjustment" and "coping" may be continually re-negotiated. Alongside this recent qualitative work on amputation and prosthesis use, I have presented a series of papers (Murray 2004, 2005, 2008, 2009) arising from a project designed to explore the embodied experience, personal and social meanings of being a prosthesis user for persons with amputation or congenital limb deficiency. In contrast to the explicit questions and focus on adjustment and coping in the above qualitative studies, my own research has a broader focus on the experience and the meaning of limb loss or absence and prosthesis use, which enabled the production of more spontaneous accounts in which these topics were implicated. The research outcomes from this project highlight the subtlety and complexity of how such persons cope or adjust in ways obscured by the more prevalent quantitative literature on these topics. Within the remainder of this chapter, I provide a narrative summary of this work (the reader is referred to the above papers for additional methodological details and data excerpts).

6.2 Study Background

The project summarised here obtained qualitative data via 35 semi-structured interviews conducted via a mix of face-to-face ($n=14$) and email ($n=21$) interviews, along with the collection of electronically stored communication between participants on two computer forums dedicated to issues of amputation, congenital limb absence and prosthesis use. Sixteen interviewees were male, 19 female. Twenty-seven of these had limb loss (24 of a lower limb; 3 upper-limb). Eight participants had congenital limb absence (four of a lower limb; four upper-limb). The age range for the whole of the sample was 16–75.

The primary data were analysed using Interpretative Phenomenological Analysis (IPA), an established qualitative method in the fields of health, social, counselling and clinical psychology (Smith 2004). The approach has its ontological roots within phenomenology, symbolic interactionism, and hermeneutics and, as a result of these influences, particular emphasis is placed on capturing and exploring the meanings that participants assign to experiences in order to gain an insider's perspective on the area of research interest. The approach also recognises the central, interpretative role of the researcher in analysing and making sense of these experiences. More detail on how analysis proceeds for this approach, along with further data excerpts can be found in the earlier cited studies.

The following is a summation of the material to be found in the aforementioned work. Table 6.1 provides further detail (including indicative data excerpts) of the main themes identified for each of the following domains to be discussed: the embodied experience, personal and social meanings of prosthesis use.

6.3 Embodied Experience

Following on from either limb loss or having congenital limb deficiency, participants described becoming familiar with a prosthetic for the first time, or with a replacement prosthetic, as a process of physical and psychological adjustment to a change in sensory information. Such an adjustment was an on-going activity, in which the body and prosthesis were continually changing, with periods of "good" and "bad" fits. Both the body and the prosthetic needed to be regulated in order to achieve a working partnership. For instance, a controlled diet was often seen as necessary to prevent changes in the shape of a residual limb, or to avoid "overloading" a prosthetic. Similarly, prostheses required good maintenance. The work to achieve this often appeared considerable, but was apparently swallowed up in routines that became automatic, requiring little thought, and, as such, allowed for smooth prosthesis use.

Prosthesis users provided accounts of the changing nature of their use over time, which gave some indication of the temporal dimension involved in the embodiment of a prosthetic limb. One aspect of this changing experience was the attention and awareness that was given to prosthesis use. Participants reported an initial period where prosthesis use required a great deal of thought, periods of exasperation, but a gradual decrease in the amount of attention or awareness of the prosthetic in use over time.

With practice and continued use participants spoke of the increasing "naturalness" of prosthesis use, and a decreased amount of concentration needed for this activity. Following a prolonged training period, as well as a period of everyday use, walking with a prosthetic could, for those with acquired limb loss, resemble the intuitive nature of walking as experienced pre-amputation. Despite a need to consciously think about the position of their legs before commencing to walk, once in movement they could "just walk".

Table 6.1 Summary of the main thematic areas (domains) and the themes within each (domain themes) arising from the study

Theme domains	Themes within each domain	Example data excerpts (numbered excerpts correspond to the numbered theme titles in the middle column)
Embodied experience (Murray 2004)	1. Adjusting to a prosthetic 2. The balance of the body 3. Awareness of the prosthesis 4. The knowing body 5. The phantom becomes the prosthesis: extending the body 6. The prosthesis as tool or corporeal structure	1. Fitting a dead thing to your live body is and always will be an imperfect process. The most critical thing is establishing a good fit. Unfortunately your body will change over time, so a good fit today may not feel as good tomorrow, then it will feel great the next day. The body changes in subtle ways that only those that wear artificial limbs can imagine. 5. Well, to me it is as if, though I have not got my lower arm, it is as though I have got it and it is [the prosthesis] part of me now. It is as though I have got two hands, two arms.
Personal meanings (Murray 2009)	1. Dreams and realities: enabling prostheses 2. Being like everybody else: the meanings of cosmesis 3. Passing, telling and getting away with it: disguising prosthesis use	1. My physical therapist said yesterday that I can start wearing the prosthesis 8 h a day. This means that I will be able to wear it [and go back] to work. A BIG (REALLY BIG) step along the road to recovery. 2. It makes me, the look of it makes me feel half way normal. It does, when I am wearing my arm, it makes me feel half way human. I am not an odd bod.
Social meanings (Murray 2005)	1. Prosthesis use and social rituals 2. Being a leper: reactions of others 3. Social meanings of concealment and disclosure 4. Feelings and experiences regarding romantic and sexual relationships	2. I have some friends and they just can not accept that I have got this problem, that I have got this leg. And I went away on holiday, with my friends last year. And I knew that these other friends were going to be there. I would not go in the wheelchair; I completely cut all my groin because of the friction of wearing it all the time. I was in a mess. Because I would not let this group of people see me without a leg on. 3. I prefer people to get to know me first before, you know, it is like the old saying they see the wheelchair before the person. Well I have always been the other way round, I want people to know me, if I can, before they know about my disability.

Occasionally, necessary routines "brought it back" or made the prosthesis user aware of their artificial limb, such as when rising from a chair and having to check the position of a prosthetic foot before beginning to walk. However, for much of the time, a practised prosthesis user could experience intuitive, pre-reflective use.

A range of activities or phenomena were cited by participants as occasions when an increased awareness of a prosthetic was experienced, such as activities which required increased physical exertion. Here, different forms of awareness were discussed – many of which could also be true of awareness of anatomical limbs. Occasionally, participants explicitly used their anatomical limbs as direct comparisons when discussing awareness of their prosthesis. As such, the instances cited did not differ greatly to general awareness of physical extremities.

A further issue to emerge related to the knowledge about corporeal structure that an artificial limb could embody and make available to prosthesis users. For instance, Rachel, an older woman with congenital limb deficiency, recounted an attempt earlier in her life to learn how to play the piano. On one particular week she had forgotten to take her left prosthetic hand with her, and her tutor asked her to "just do the right hand, but think where the left hand would be". As Rachel explained, without the presence of her prosthetic limb, "I could not think left handed".

It became evident that the prosthetic hand was able to provide Rachel with knowledge that is usually corporeal. In this manner, using a prosthetic becomes a form of knowing – an understanding which is achieved practically and corporeally. Rachel described both the limits and the potentiality of a prosthetic hand. While she was unable to perform complex motor acts with the prosthetic, relatively simple activities, such as holding a hymnbook in church, were made "knowable" to her by virtue of the prosthesis. While this was an experience recounted by a number of participants, it was all the more interesting that this was often the experience of participants who had congenital limb absence, and could not only describe the experience of having an artificial limb re-design the "natural" topography of their body, but also imbue the implicit knowledge which is usually embodied.

Interviews with participants often revealed senses in which the prosthetic limb was experienced as part of the phenomenal body. Such experiences were frequently evident in their descriptions of phantom limb phenomena, and of direct assertions of the prosthesis feeling "part of" them. The phantom limb phenomenon is a common feature of amputation (see Chaps. 9–11 in this volume). Typically, people with amputations report feeling as if their amputated limb is "still there". The experience of a phantom limb as part of the phenomenal body and its potential to positively or negatively impact upon prosthesis experience was apparent in research interviews. Sometimes the phenomenal topography of the phantom limb was so distorted so that it was near impossible for it to assume the same position as the prosthetic limb. However, often the phantom and the prosthetic were interlaced into a phenomenal corporeal structure, such as when walking.

Interviewees reported the combinative effect of prosthesis and phantom limb as negating a feeling of bodily loss. The spatial and topographical correspondence of the phantom and prosthetic facilitated function, namely the use of a prosthetic was aided by the sensory experience of the phantom. However, for other participants, such an experience, where the phantom and prosthetic limb entwine, was a temporary one. A high leg amputation, for instance, meant that an increased amount of concentration was necessary for effective prosthesis use, and this unravelled the feeling that the amputated limb had been "replaced".

For many participants with amputations or with congenital limb absence, a prosthetic was often capable of being experienced as "part of" the body. Here, the prosthetic was incorporated into bodily space so that it too is included in those areas which feel intimately our own. The sense of ownership and spatiality that accompanies corporeal structures is extended to the prosthetic device. In such circumstances, a sense of completeness is engendered by the prosthesis. The prosthetic itself was experienced by some respondents as a source of sensorial experience. For example when, although in a "cruder" manner than before the amputation, participants reported feeling the texture of the ground on the sole of their phantom foot whilst walking (see Murray 2008 for a discussion of this experience in relation to phenomenological theory regarding tool use).

Such descriptions from participants convey the experience whereby a prosthetic is incorporated into bodily space and becomes a sentient extension of the body. However, not all participants described their prosthesis as an extension of their body. While for some using a prosthetic was an emotionally charged affair, in which a sense of completeness and regained abilities were engendered, for others this remained a practical issue. In this manner, artificial limbs were viewed as tools that, in the case of artificial legs, provided imperfect solutions to mobility problems.

Clearly, prosthesis users differ in their embodied experience of prosthesis use. While many such users report a feeling of a prosthetic as part of the phenomenal body, for others the prosthetic remains a valuable enabling tool without this experiential aspect.

6.4 Personal Meanings

Despite the aforementioned variation in the degree to which a prosthetic felt part of the phenomenal body, beginning to use a prosthetic limb with some success was generally of deep personal significance for participants. This was particularly apparent for participants with lower-limb amputations, for whom – following the trauma of amputation, and a loss of some bodily abilities – beginning to use a prosthetic leg, and hence to be mobile again, was often interpreted as a key moment in "getting" their "life back again".

A sense of "recovery" when beginning to use a prosthetic limb was often spoken about. For instance, a prosthetic leg was readily associated with mobility, and in enabling the expression of the self in significant activities. One such activity that was highly valued was paid employment. As such, being able to walk was closely associated with being able to return to work, to regain, or "get back" a working identity. The profound sense that a prosthetic limb could be a "life-enhancing tool" was apparent. Here, a deeply held desire to be able to walk once more was seen as possible through the long process of learning to use a prosthetic leg. As such, possible alternatives, such as a wheelchair, were not considered as adequate alternatives.

Rather than discussing the failings or benefits of prostheses in isolation, participants tended to make favourable comparisons with able-bodied people. Here, the limitations of prostheses were often compared to the limitations of able-bodied people in general. In this manner, participants emphasised the positive aspects of their artificial leg – what it enabled. While prosthetic limbs were often conceived of as "imperfect", "poor substitutes" or merely tools, the personal meanings of what such devices could enable was often profound. Desires, such as being able to wear certain shoes, to dance, or to "run around" with one's children, were often fulfilled for participants by using a prosthetic leg.

Along with enabling participation in both seemingly mundane, and less mundane, activities, the significance of appearing and living life "like everybody does" and to be treated "like everyone else" were of profound importance. Prosthesis use thus allowed independent travel, and participation in social activities. Prostheses were considered not only as enabling devices, but participants often conceived their prosthesis as central to their personal (and social) identity. Prostheses enabled participation in work and in personally and socially valued activities, such as driving.

Interviewees recounted very personal experiences, such as family relationships and involvement in paid employment, to illustrate how using a prosthetic limb had enabled particular activities with personal significance. Here, the importance of a prosthetic limb was recounted in participants' historical biographical narratives. For example, one participant recounted the role his prosthesis had played in courtship, activities as a father with his son, and so on. As such, participants "grew into" their prostheses over and through important life events.

The value of "cosmesis" in a prosthetic limb – such as a skin-coloured cosmetic cover to conceal the working components of an artificial limb, or close visual approximation of a limb's characteristics (including, in some cases, veins, hair and realistic looking digits and nails) – was frequently described as of personal value to participants. A realistic-looking, but non-functional, passive limb was sometimes preferred to a more functional, but less aesthetically pleasing, prosthetic limb (for example, the upper-limb hook).

The desire to appear bodily complete was compelling for many participants, even when the process of learning to use a prosthetic limb was described as a painful and arduous one. Participants talked of their initial (and in some cases enduring) dislike, even hate, towards their prosthesis. However, despite this, the profound sense of normalcy that using a prosthetic limb instilled was still evident. This is demonstrated in the account of one female, an upper-limb prosthesis user, who described the tension that existed for her between the negative and positive aspects of her prosthesis. In particular, her prosthesis was discussed as a device which could maintain her humanness ("half way human"), which in turn prevented her, quite literally, from being seen to have an "odd" body.

However, not all participants considered cosmesis as important, and a number of participants actually conveyed a distaste for the use of cosmetic limbs in general, seeing such use as indicative of an inability to "deal with" limb loss/absence, or even as conspiring in an oppressive climate in which people with limb loss/absence were pressured to conform, or be ashamed of their prosthesis use. Participants who expressed these views were more likely to focus on the functional, or pragmatic, merits and uses of prostheses rather than any cosmetic or aesthetic benefit. Ambivalence or disapproval towards cosmetic limbs was often (but not exclusively) expressed by those users whose movement with a prosthetic limb was noticeable to others. For instance, participants referred to a poor walking gait as revealing to others and able to draw "stares".

In contrast to those participants who sought cosmesis, a hiding or disguising of amputation, a sizeable number of participants were militant in an approach that might be termed "prosthetic limb display". Here, participants displayed their amputation, limb absence and prosthesis use as a method of defiance, resistance, and to challenge notions of disability. As such "prosthetic display" held profound personal significance and meaning to self and social identity, and was part of the politicisation of disability. Rather than trying to avoid the stares of others, these participants recognised that people would stare, and therefore accentuated the visibility of prosthesis use. Such participants often celebrated the design and use of prosthetic limbs, with any embarrassment experienced not being due to the public visibility of their prosthesis use, but to those occasions when their prostheses did not perform as expected.

Linked with the meaning of cosmesis, the research identified issues relating to the personal meaning of disguising prosthesis use. "Disguising" was often spoken of as an activity that might, for instance, involve the strategic wearing of clothes in order to conceal limb loss/absence and prosthesis use. However, while the possibility of concealing prosthesis use was available to adept users, such as those with lower-limb amputations who walked well and had prostheses high in cosmesis, for other participants "disguising" prosthesis use was considered unworkable due to a conspicuous walking gait or obvious prosthesis. In contrast to the disguising practices of some interviewees, such as the types of clothes worn, these participants did not adopt such strategies, but wore their clothes of choice, such as shorts or short skirts, regardless of whether they made their limb loss/absence and prosthesis use more apparent to others.

Participants' ability to manage personal information relating to concealment and disclosure allowed many prosthesis users to "pass" as able-bodied. However, such ability often had a significant impact upon self expression and personal development; participants sometimes regretted the amount of time and effort they had invested in learning to "walk perfectly" and reflected it would have been better for their own healing if they had been more exposed and forced to address rather than hide their limb loss. Being able to "pass" was often conceived as an activity that was almost deceptive, such as when participants spoke of "getting away with it". However, this activity of "passing" was sometimes performed for the benefit of others, for whom participants felt it might be uncomfortable to be faced with the reality of their situation.

Participants often experienced dilemmas of how and when to reveal information regarding prosthesis use. If an inopportune moment arose, participants were faced with a decision as to whether to reveal this information then or not (such as being asked to run to catch a bus by someone who did not know they had had an amputation). Not doing so had implications for a person's self-image, with regards to whether they were being deceptive. Therefore, participants would recount awkward situations, in which their insistence not to "deny" their prosthesis use could have embarrassing repercussions. However, the value which prosthesis users imputed to being able to "not-show" their limb loss/absence and prosthesis use was apparent. One participant explained that a combination of gait and prosthetic limb design meant that many people hardly "noticed", which therefore made him "one of the fortunate invisible amputees".

In contrast, for other prosthesis users the concealment of limb loss/absence through prosthesis use was considered an important method of combating prejudice. The invisibility of limb absence afforded by prosthesis use enabled the formation of relationships which were in no manner predicated upon or discouraged by the fact of limb absence or "disability".

6.5 Social Meanings

Participants related a range of social meanings surrounding and implicated in their prosthesis use. The ability to accomplish what are usually taken-for-granted embodied capabilities by those without limb loss or deficiencies were recounted as of profound importance – such as eating with a knife and fork, which for one participant, Rachel, was enabled by a specially designed prosthesis that had a fork attachment. Similarly, in Western cultures, the loss of a right hand means that the person is no longer able to shake hands in the socially accepted manner, whereas the loss of the left hand prevents them from wearing their wedding ring on the "correct" hand (Dise-Lewis 1989). A prosthetic limb, then, may be able to restore some of these rudimentary customs in which the body is routinely and socially deployed.

In a discussion of Goffman's work regarding the body, Shilling (1993) argues that "encounters" are important aspects of social life in which people are concerned to act out specific roles (such as the above participant's competent diner-in-a-restaurant). However, in order to be convincing in these roles, they must abide by the "corporeal rules" that proscribe such encounters. In the above example, these corporeal rules include the use of a knife and fork to eat a meal. In addition to being able to eat in public in a socially acceptable manner, the prosthetically enabled ability to eat with a knife and fork for this participant also meant that she could escape a form of infantalization. For instance, she described how she had taught her own child how to eat with a knife and fork, and so the ability to do this was readily associated by the participant with maturing into adulthood. Therefore, prosthesis use could help to maintain an identity as a competent adult. As such, we can appreciate how prostheses allow people with limb loss or congenital limb absence to take part in culturally and socially valued activities that are predicated upon able-bodiedness.

How other people actively encountered and reacted to the fact of prosthesis use was of extreme social significance to participants. People's responses could be experienced as offensive, such as when they distanced themselves by physically moving away, or they could be intrusive such as when strangers asked direct questions regarding participants' limb loss/absence and prosthesis use.

As well as providing accounts of the reactions of strangers to their condition, participants also spoke of friends' reactions. These reactions were frequently negative, with some close friends avoiding all contact. However, not all responses were negative. Participants were frequently mistaken in their expectations of how friends would react. Here some respondents emphasized the prosthesis user's role in being "fine" about it, so that others could be too. In addition to being "fine" about it, occasionally it was argued that prosthesis users themselves had some responsibility to "demonstrate" their capabilities in public, and their right to be in public life. This accords with Radley (1993), who suggested that the implied stigma of illness (which can also apply to disabilities) necessitates the use of a number of measures to hide or modify differences in order for an individual to be considered a fully capable participant in social life.

Kelly and Field (1996) argue that to be recognized as capable social actors it is necessary to demonstrate one's capacity in bodily management. Therefore, a "competent" appearance is very important for people with disabilities or illness, such as with Charmaz's (1995) participants who made a great deal of effort to appear well and able-bodied so as not to lose the support of employers and colleagues, or even their jobs. For some participants, knowing that others were uncomfortable with their limb loss/absence and prosthesis use was sufficient for them to "cater" for others. In this regard, one participant told how, although she would prefer not to wear her prosthesis when at home, would do so in the presence of her brother who could not "accept it". This could be upsetting inasmuch as it revealed the inability of close friends to "accept" limb loss. On occasions when such people were present, prostheses were often worn for their benefit.

In so far as prosthesis users wore their artificial limb at those times they would rather not, they contributed to what Goffman (1963) termed the "bureaucratization of the spirit". This is the result of a large amount of time when individuals are required to be "on stage", producing consistent performances during social encounters. Goffman suggested individuals needed relaxation within "back-regions" where they could indulge in "creature releases". Similarly, participants described how they would take off their prosthesis when alone, an act which appeared to be a "creature release" for them.

The way in which wearing and not wearing a prosthetic could impact upon and shape the social identity of an individual was often stark. Wearing a prosthetic could enable a user to be accepted as an equal, with no special treatment or fuss. However, when a prosthetic was not used, but perhaps a wheelchair or crutches instead, then the same people might react quite differently, emphasizing the difference and the disabled status of the prosthesis user. Similarly, Gardner (1986) has written about the tendency for some people to see the use of a wheelchair as an "implied petition" for help. In this way, helpful strangers may perceive wheelchair users as less competent than they actually are.

The social meanings of concealment of prosthesis use, and the ability to control disclosure of this information, were often discussed by participants. Prosthesis use was often conceived of as a practice that helped maintain a "secret identity", namely one of able-bodiedness. However, prosthesis use itself was not enough to supply such an "identity" and various strategies and regimens were often necessary in order to achieve this. For instance, one participant in the U.S. Army Reserve kept his limb loss a secret during a 2-week summer camp by showering while his colleagues slept, always wearing long trousers and nightwear, and only "popping off" his artificial leg while in his sleeping bag.

Such experiences of participants' prosthesis use in this research can be compared with those of other people with a disability or chronic illness. For instance, some people with disability or chronic illness portray public identities that downplay or deny the current impact of their condition on their day-to-day lives (Charmaz 1995). They may need to expend a great deal of time and energy in order to make this perception believable to others. In my own work with prosthesis users, the fact that other people could not "tell" that participants had limb loss/absence and used prosthetics, and their surprise when they discovered this information, was deeply pleasurable for many participants. However, in addition to this, to the extent that a prosthetic, in partnership with strategies of concealment, enabled the safeguarding of this information, participants felt able to live fulfilling and independent lives.

The ability to conceal, and control disclosure of information regarding limb loss/absence and prosthesis use by virtue of its low visibility provided some tensions of its own. On occasions when people "find out" this could prove embarrassing to the person concerned when they "drag[ged] something out" with which they were uncomfortable. While the invisibility of limb absence, made possible by prosthesis use, was recognized by many participants, this invisibility could also make it difficult to broach the subject with others. Participants sometimes explained how the concealment of their prosthesis became a way of being able to "get yourself across as a person" to other people, so that they "coped" with the fact of the prosthesis at a later time. Therefore, the potential invisibility afforded by prosthesis use was conceived as useful in allowing relationships to be forged which were not predicated upon, or hindered by, the fact of limb absence. In this manner, the "true" person could be known without "disability" impacting first on such a relationship.

The ability to conceal bodily difference, then, was seen by many participants as pivotal in avoiding stigma, with the social identities of disabled people so often hinging upon the public availability of this information. Participants drawn from the on-line discussion groups were often involved in discussions regarding the identities of those prosthesis users who could and those who could not conceal their limb loss/absence. Here, the ability to conceal this information was used to contest what a "real" amputee was. As such, the exchanges are informative of just how important some prosthesis users view the ability to control concealment and disclosure in having an identity of "amputee" or "disabled".

6.6 General Discussion

Within this chapter the embodied experience, personal and social meanings of prosthesis use have been presented. Participants' accounts enable a fuller understanding of how they attempted to adjust and cope with limb loss or absence and prosthesis use. In what follows below I summarise these findings from each of the areas and relate them to implications for health professionals working with this population

6.6.1 Embodied Experience

Here, I have elaborated the embodied perceptual experience of prosthesis use, including the issue of if, and to what extent, a prosthetic limb can be incorporated into the sensorial architecture of the person's body. The themes presented reflect the possibility that under certain circumstances a prosthetic can be transformed from an "extracorporeal structure" into a corporeal one. The experience of a phantom limb, whereby many amputees feel as if the anatomical limb is still intact and present in its usual place, often played a large part in enabling the incorporation of a prosthetic into the phenomenal body of participants, such as when the prosthetic limb was experienced as part of the phenomenal body, with the phantom and the prosthetic interlacing into a phenomenal corporeal structure.

Participants reported that a decreased awareness of a prosthetic accompanied practiced use. This is not to say that all prosthesis users have this experience, in fact some did not and described their prostheses merely as practical aids. However, the experience of a prosthetic as part of the phenomenal body was a common occurrence. One interesting aspect of this research is that not only did prosthesis users experience this, but the prosthesis became a source of perceptual information as well as actionable possibility as part of the prosthesis user's phenomenological body boundaries. One important aspect of this work is that, whereas previous research has found that the increased physical effort associated with prosthesis use as well as discomfort experienced when wearing a prosthetic often leads to rejection of artificial limbs, the present research suggests that these experiences may be negated with perseverance. That is, the often cited reasons for the rejection of prostheses are frequently part of the initial experiences of "successful" prosthesis users also who, unlike those who "reject" their prosthesis, persist with using their artificial limbs to find that these negative experiences give way to a more natural pre-reflective use of their artificial limbs.

The above may, in part, explain the association between level of prosthesis use and satisfaction of amputees towards their prosthesis: time plus use knits together prosthesis satisfaction and pre-reflective prosthesis use. Once again, this is not to argue that all prosthesis users would come to have such pre-reflective prosthesis use; indeed, many amputees, for instance, will not have the physical strength (particularly if they are elderly) or a residual limb which affords such an outcome.

However, this present research does raise the possibility that many people who could benefit from prosthesis use simply do not persevere to the point where these benefits could be realized.

These findings have implications for rehabilitation. First, the data presented herein reinforce the importance of achieving a good "fit" between prosthesis socket and residual limb in initial consultations between limb wearers and prosthetists. However, this "good fit" needs to be recognized as a temporal and continual process, which requires the involvement of prosthesis users, for instance in diet, activity and prosthetic limb maintenance. If these considerations are not effectively communicated to new limb users, or if such responsibility is shunned, then the possibility of rejection of the limb in everyday life can be expected to increase.

A second implication is that the training of persons to use artificial limbs should emphasize the long-term process involved, for instance, in gaining effective balance and walking gait with the aid of a prosthetic. The use of an artificial limb is not intuitive to begin with, nor does such use initially feel "natural". However, participants in the research reported here stressed the process of "adjustment" to using a prosthetic in which there was a "natural" switch and "subconscious compensation" to changes in weight distribution and body balance following amputation and subsequent prosthesis use. It is likely that currently many prosthesis users abandon such use before adjustment takes place in the mistaken belief that their experience will never change. These implications suggest the need to sufficiently motivate potential prosthesis users in the period between an experience of prosthesis use as unnatural and wieldy to one of pre-reflective, natural use. It should be noted that while the reported research here is informative in this regard, it cannot provide an approximation of when in the rehabilitative process such a change should take place. There are a number of considerations which would need to be examined, including amputation site, type of prosthesis used, the amount of time that a limb is used for and for which activities, as well as demographic and psycho-social variables of the prosthesis user. Therefore more statistically based approaches would be better suited to address this issue.

Finally, it is important to note that two broad forms of prosthesis experience can be characterized from this research: one in which the prosthesis was experienced as a corporeal structure; and one in which it was viewed as a tool. Both of these experiences characterized different persons who were nevertheless "successful" prosthesis users. While future work may be able to explore the psychosocial correlates of these experiences, it is nonetheless the case that persons with these differing experiences were able to enjoy the benefits imbued by prosthesis use.

6.6.2 *Personal Meanings*

Prior research has emphasised how non-use of a prosthetic limb leads to the restriction of everyday activities (Williamson 1995). The research reported here had a concern with those people who use a prosthetic limb following amputation or congenital limb absence, and has considered the meanings of active prosthesis use. What is apparent is how and why prosthesis use not only contributes to a more active lifestyle, but also why this is so important for participants. Research participants valued the benefits (which might be considered mundane or taken-for-granted by able-bodied persons) afforded by a prosthetic limb, where the personal meanings of what such devices could enable was often profound. Desires of being able to wear shoes, to dance, or to "run around" were often fulfilled for participants. The significance of appearing and living life "like everybody does" and to be treated "like everyone else" were apparent, allowed independent travel, participation in social activities, and as such prostheses were of profound importance.

The key goal in the rehabilitation of the lower-limb amputee is the regaining of mobility, with a high number of studies using this as the dominant measure of successful rehabilitation (Stein and Walley 1983). However, what is lacking in these studies is the meaning of such capabilities as enabled by prosthesis use. In the present research, beginning to use a prosthetic limb with some success was of deep personal significance for participants, and was often viewed as a key moment in "getting" their "life back again". A sense of "recovery" was communicated, with a prosthetic leg being readily associated with mobility, and in reconstructing the self in significant activities, such as paid employment. Even with the first tentative steps with a prosthetic limb, many participants spoke of the good feeling of standing up once again, and of how this made them believe that walking again was a real possibility. As such, these participants spoke of the importance of their prostheses for personal identity, for maintaining independence and for being integral to important life events. Importantly, it was not mobility (which could be provided with a wheelchair) per se that participants wished for (as implied in previous research), but for actual "normal" walking.

One aspect of prosthesis use that was important for many participants was cosmesis. A variety of meanings surrounded the use of prosthetic limbs with cosmetic covers, and realistic features. For some cosmesis was paramount, while others emphasized comfort, and others stressed the importance of having a prosthetic limb that was functional. When choices had to be made between limbs that were aesthetically pleasing, and having a limb that was more functional, participants were generally divided (in terms of actual numbers) between those who opted for cosmesis and those who opted for function. However, some participants had changed their opinions on this issue over time. For example, many participants with a recent amputation were concerned to hide their limb loss through use of a prosthetic limb. For some of these, this anxiety subsided and prostheses became to be viewed much more as enabling devices.

The suggestion that prostheses are often rejected because they are not attractive to look at (Millstein et al. 1986) finds some support in this research: a realistic-looking passive limb was sometimes preferred to a more functional, but less aesthetically pleasing, prosthetic limb (for example the upper-limb hook). However, cosmesis alone was not sufficient; those participants whose movement with a prosthetic limb was telling to others often conceived of a cosmetic prosthesis as able to draw "stares" and therefore not "making a difference".

With regard to the variety of responses to cosmetic limbs by participants, we can consider the context of "normalisation". Two meanings or uses of the term "normalisation" emerge in disability literature. The first refers to attempts by the person to adjust to, and fit in with, wider society (Phillips 1985), and, is seen as an expression of an internalisation of socially devalued personal identities. The decision by some participants in the present research to use prosthetic limbs visually redolent of anatomical limbs is arguably an example of this, along with attempts to disguise their prosthesis use.

The strategic use of clothing was one technique by which such detail could be hidden from others' awareness. Such practice can be considered in relation to research by Kaiser et al. (1985, 1987) who discussed the role of clothing in the management of appearances by persons with physical disabilities. Kaiser et al. found that most disabled persons strived to appear as normative as possible through their clothing choices, using a variety of techniques to conceal or deflect attention away from their disabilities, which they referred to as "appearance management".

The second meaning of normalisation in the disability literature is one which involves its acceptance and acknowledgement. Here, disabled people gain social success without denying their disability or internalising devalued personal identities (Phillips 1985). A decision not to use prosthetic limbs, or, as with some participants in the present research, not to use prosthetic limbs designed to "disguise" their artificial nature, might be considered an example of this (Frank 1988).

Such participants deliberately chose prostheses that cosmetically did not resemble non-amputees' bodies but which may function as such. The practice of prosthetic display described earlier can be compared favourably with the work of Gelya Frank (1988), who discussed the experiences of three adults with severe multiple congenital limb deficiencies.

For these individuals "self display" was a strategy for self-empowerment in which the primary focus was the experience of the person with disabilities rather than reactions of people who are "normal". As Frank argues, by insisting on being visible as people with disabilities, they appeared to reject the stigmatization of their physical appearance. Part of this visibility comes from choosing not to use prostheses.

Frank continues that people with visible disabilities, and who choose to place themselves in public situations, and identify as disabled, go beyond "covering" and "passing", and as such these behaviours can be elaborated and articulated into strategies for dealing with stigma and enabling empowerment. However, interestingly, in the research reported here, some participants were able to adopt the functional benefits of prostheses in a manner which still allowed "self display" and hence the rejection of stigma.

Within this chapter the personal meanings of prosthesis use have been presented. The value participants with limb loss and with congenital limb absence placed upon artificial limbs for practical accomplishments, the management of personal information, and the maintenance of identities has been highlighted. This research reveals a deeper understanding of why and how prosthesis use for many people enriches their quality of life and facilitates adapting and coping processes. It also explicates the experience, management and negation of stigma by such persons. Taken together, the themes presented herein lend support to the view that prosthesis use can greatly increase the psychological health and well being of people with limb loss and absence. The outcomes of the present research suggest that it is important for health professionals involved in prosthesis users' medical care and personal welfare to recognise the need for (and to make possible) the maintenance of valued identities and the self management of their disability status.

6.6.3 Social Meanings

In the research reported here, participants recounted the often negative responses of others towards their limb loss/absence and prosthesis use which were of extreme social significance to them. These experiences included offensive and intrusive behaviours. Such experiences impacted highly upon participants' social identities. Such social reactions might be expected to lead such persons to limit their social contact. In Goffman's (1963) seminal work on stigma, he argued that the perception and meanings of bodies are constituted, in part, during social interaction. The socially acceptable management of the body is important in a person's self-identity. While the management of bodily performance in social interaction tends to proceed, for most people, most of the time, in an unproblematic manner, for people with disabilities their ability to achieve this is often compromised. Therefore, particularly when such a disability as amputation or congenital limb absence is highly visible, withdrawal from social contact becomes the means by which negative social encounters are avoided.

However, while the avoidance of social contact minimizes the problem of social stigmatization, other problems surround this. Such persons' level of depression has been found to increase as their level of activity and satisfaction with social contacts decrease (Williamson et al. 1994). Higher levels of depression have been linked to lower levels of social support (Rybarczyk et al. 1992), higher levels of social discomfort (Rybarczyk et al. 1992) and higher levels of perceived social stigma (Rybarczyk et al. 1995).

The person's perceived control over their disability has also been found to predict lower scores on a depression scale and higher scores on a self-esteem scale (Dunn 1996). One way that participants overcame social withdrawal and its associated problems was to become skilled in impression management, often using prostheses to conceal disability and hence be able to make decisions for themselves about when and to whom to disclose this information.

Such an approach required skilful, natural use of a prosthesis, the strategic use of clothing and daily routines that combined to make prosthesis use a secret identity. Whereas prior research has found that satisfaction with, and use of, a prosthesis is positively associated with increased social integration and an absence of emotional problems (Ham and Cotton 1991), the present research would suggest that it is, in part, ease of prosthesis use, and its ability to conceal limb loss/absence and ward off social stigmatization that enables social integration and the reduction of emotional problems surrounding such disability.

The way in which wearing and not wearing a prosthetic could impact upon and show the social identity of an individual was often stark. Even when a prosthetic user was known as such to sets of individuals, the presence or absence of a prosthetic could invoke entirely different sets of behaviours, and as such were important in defining a person's social identity. As such, the prosthetic was part of the presentation of self to others, integral to the day-to-day praxis of the body, embedded and embodied as they were in social situations in which bodily competency, the ability "to handle" their bodies, was crucial to a sense of self-identity.

To conclude, the meanings and experiences as revealed in the present research demonstrate the folly of attending solely to the physical properties of a prosthetic. For instance, while Millstein et al. (1986) reasonably suggest that a prosthetic should be comfortable, functional and cosmetic, in the present research prostheses were found to be used despite sometimes not being one or more of these. Indeed, while there has been a preponderance of literature that focuses either on the physical properties of the prosthesis (e.g. its usefulness for particular tasks (Stein and Walley 1983) and its functional reliability (Balance et al. 1989), or the psychological problems of potential wearers (Friedmann 1978), perhaps the strongest contribution the present research makes is the recognition and elaboration of the social role of the prosthesis and how this is central to how participants are continually engaged in processes of adapting and coping.

6.7 Conclusion

I began this chapter by highlighting a pervasive structured, quantitative approach to issues of adjustment and coping to amputation and prosthesis use, and how recent qualitative work has added to this approach and knowledge base. This work, along with my own reported here, enables a broader and deeper understanding of how coping or adjustment is actually experienced and achieved, as well as a more sophisticated conceptualisation of what it is these terms refer to. Through examining the meanings and experiences of the material circumstances of those with acquired limb loss and congenital limb absence or deficiencies, it becomes possible to better inform and develop the range of services, which are provided by a broad group of health professionals to meet the needs of this group.

References

Balance R, Wilson B, Harder JA (1989) Factors affecting myoelectric prosthetic limb use and wearing patterns in the juvenile unilateral below-elbow amputee. Can J Occup Ther 56(3):132–137

Charmaz K (1995) The body, identity, and self: adapting to impairment. Sociol Q 36(4):657–680

Desmond DM (2007) Coping, affective distress and psychosocial adjustment among people with traumatic upper limb amputations. J Psychosom Res 62(1):15–21

Dise-Lewis JE (1989) Psychological adaptation to limb loss. In: Atkins DJ, Meyer RH (eds) Comprehensive management of the upper-limb amputee. Springer, New York, pp 165–172

Dunn DS (1996) Well-being following amputation: salutary effects of positive meaning, optimism and control. Rehabil Psychol 41(4):285–302

Frank G (1986) On embodiment: a case of congenital limb deficiency in American culture. Cult Med Psychiatry 10:189–219

Frank G (1988) Beyond stigma: visibility and self-empowerment of persons with congenital limb deficiencies. J Soc Issues 44(1):95–115

Friedmann LW (1978) The psychological rehabilitation of the amputee. Charles C. Thomas, Springfield, IL

Gallagher P, McLachlan M (2001) Adjustment to an artificial limb: a qualitative perspective. J Health Psychol 6(1):85–100

Gardner C (1986) Public aid. Urban Life 15:37–69

Goffman E (1963) Stigma: notes on the management of spoiled identity. Prentice-Hall, Englewood Cliffs, NJ

Ham RO, Cotton LT (1991) Limb amputation: from aetiology to rehabilitation. Chapman & Hall, London

Horgan O, MacLachlan M (2004) Psychosocial adjustment to lower limb amputation: a review. Disabil Rehabil 26(14–15):837–850

Kaiser SB, Freeman CM, Wingate SB (1985) Stigmata and negotiated outcomes: management of appearance by persons with physical disabilities. Deviant Behav 6(2):205–224

Kaiser SB, Wingate SB, Freeman CM, Chandler JL (1987) Acceptance of physical disability and attitudes toward personal appearance. Rehabil Psychol 32(1):51–58

Kelly MP, Field D (1996) Medical sociology, chronic illness and the body. Sociol Health Illn 18(2):241–257

Millstein SG, Heger H, Hunter GA (1986) Prosthetic use in adult and upper limb amputees: a comparison of the body powered and electrically powered prostheses. Prosthet Orthot Int 10:27–34

Murray CD (2004) An interpretative phenomenological analysis of the embodiment of artificial limbs. Disabil Rehabil 26(16):963–973

Murray CD (2005) The social meanings of prosthesis use. J Health Psychol 10(3):425–441

Murray CD (2008) Embodiment and prosthetics. In: Gallagher P, Desmond D, MacLachlan M (eds) Psychoprosthetics: state of the knowledge. Springer, London, pp 119–130

Murray CD (2009) The personal meanings of prosthesis use. Disabil Rehabil 31(7):573–581

Oaksford K, Frude N, Cuddihy R (2005) Positive coping and stress-related psychological growth following lower limb amputation. Rehabil Psychol 50(3):266–277

Phillips MJ (1985) "Try harder": the experience of disability and the dilemma of normalization. J Soc Sci 22(4):45–47

Radley A (1993) The role of metaphor in adjustment to chronic illness. In: Radley A (ed.) Worlds of illness: biographical and cultural perspectives on health and disease. Routledge, London, 109–123

Rybarczyk BD, Nyenhuis DL, Nicholas JJ, Schulz R, Alioto RJ, Blair C (1992) Social discomfort and depression in a sample of adults with leg amputations. Arch Phys Med Rehabil 73(12):1169–1173

Rybarczyk BD, Nyenhuis DL, Nicholas JJ, Cash SM, Kaiser J (1995) Body image, perceived social stigma, and the prediction of psychosocial adjustment to leg amputation. Rehabil Psychol 40(2):95–110

Saradjian A, Thompson AR, Datta D (2008) The experience of men using an upper limb prosthesis following amputation: positive coping and minimizing feeling different. Disabil Rehabil 30(11):871–883

Schulz M (2009) Coping psychologically with amputation. Vasa 38(74):72–74

Shilling C (1993) The body and social theory. Sage, London

Smith JA (2004) Reflections on the development of interpretative phenomenological analysis and its contribution to qualitative research in psychology. Qual Res Psychol 1(1):39–54

Stein RB, Walley OT (1983) Functional comparison of upper extremity amputees using myoelectric and conventional prostheses. Arch Phys Med Rehabil 64:243–248

Williamson GM, Schulz R, Bridges MW, Behan AM (1994) Social and psychological factors in adjustment to limb amputation. Journal of Social Behavior and Personality 9:249–268

Williamson GM (1995) Restriction of normal activities among older amputees. J Clin Geropsychol 1:229–242

Chapter 7
Return to Work After Amputation

Helena Burger

Abstract The main objective in the rehabilitation of people following amputation is to restore or improve their functioning, which includes their return to work. People after lower or upper limb amputation have problems returning to work and working. Owing to the different functions of our lower and upper limbs, problems at work differ between both groups.

Most authors find the return to work rate to be about 66% (from 43.5 to 100% for participants after lower limb amputation and 53–100% for people after upper limb amputation). Twenty-two (22) to 67% of people after lower limb amputation retain the same occupation following amputation. Twenty (20) to 100% after upper limb amputation have to change it. Post-amputation jobs are generally more complex with a requirement for a higher level of general educational development and are physically less demanding. The return to work depends on general factors, such as age, gender and educational level; factors related to impairments and disabilities because of amputation (amputation level, multiple amputations, co-morbidity, reason for amputation, persistent stump problems, the time from the injury to obtaining a permanent prosthesis, wearing comfort of the prosthesis, walking distance and restrictions in mobility); rehabilitation; factors related to prosthesis; and factors related to work and policies (salary, higher job involvement, good support from the implementing body and the employer and social support network).

Vocational rehabilitation and counselling should become a part of rehabilitation programs for all people, who are of working age, following amputation. Better co-operation between professionals, such as rehabilitation team members, implementing bodies, company doctors and employers is necessary.

H. Burger
Institute of Rehabilitation, Ljubljana, Slovenia
e-mail: helena.burger@ir-rs.si

C. Murray (ed.), *Amputation, Prosthesis Use, and Phantom Limb Pain: An Interdisciplinary Perspective*, DOI 10.1007/978-0-387-87462-3_7,

7.1 Introduction

The main objective in the rehabilitation of people following amputation is to restore or improve their functioning, which includes their return to work. Full-time employment leads to beneficial health effects and being healthy leads to increased chances of full-time employment (Ross and Mirowskay 1995). Employment of disabled people enhances their self-esteem and reduces social isolation (Dougherty 1999). The importance of returning to work for people following amputation therefore has to be considered.

Perhaps the first article about reemployment and problems people may have at work after amputation was published in 1955 (Boynton 1955). In later years, there have been sporadic studies on this topic. Greater interest and more studies about returning to work and problems people have at work following amputation arose in the 1990s and has continued in recent years (Burger and Marinček 2007). These studies were conducted in different countries on all the five continents, the greatest number being carried out in Europe, mainly in the Netherlands and the UK (Burger and Marinček 2007).

Owing to the different functions of our lower and upper limbs, people with lower limb amputations have different activity limitations and participation restrictions compared to people with upper limb amputations. Both have problems with driving and carrying objects. People with lower limb amputations also have problems standing, walking, running, kicking, turning and stamping, whereas people with upper limb amputations have problems grasping, lifting, pushing, pulling, writing, typing, and pounding (Giridhar et al. 2001).

7.2 Lower Limb Amputation and Work

7.2.1 Successful Return to Work

The percentage of people who return to work successfully following amputation differs from study to study; these results are difficult to compare. Bruins et al. (2003) included only people who returned to work. Others reported the rate of employable age (Jones et al. 1993; Kegel et al. 1978; Nissen and Newman 1992). Schoppen et al. (2001a) included those who worked before amputation; Pohjolainen et al. (1990), only those younger than 65; Ebrahimzadeh and Rajabi (2007), people undergoing war-related amputations of the foot and ankle; Somasundaram and Renol (1998) all those who suffered amputation; whereas Atesalp et al. (1999) only those who had bilateral lower limb amputation because of landmines. The rate of employment or unemployment depends on the definition selected and varies in one single study from 71.5 to 88.4% depending on the chosen definition (Millstein et al. 1985). The reemployment rate ranges from 43.5% (Whyte and Carroll 2002) to 100% for people who suffered amputation because of a tumour (Ferrapie et al. 2003).

Most researchers found the percentage of amputees returning to work around 66% or two thirds (Curley et al. 1982; Dougherty 1999; Fisher et al. 2003; Schoppen et al. 2001a). Smith et al. (2005) found it at 66.7% for unilateral but only at 16% for bilateral amputees.

Mezghani-Masmoudi et al. (2004) report a reemployment rate of 58.3%. Additionally, they included 35.5% of amputees as taking a vocational rehabilitation program. They did not report how many were reemployed later.

Re-employment rate alone does not provide enough information. Many people only work part time following amputation. The percentage of such participants who worked part time have ranged from 34% (Schoppen et al. 2001a) to 50% (Jones et al. 1993; Livingston et al. 1994). Both studies with the highest percentage of people working part time only had a small sample (three out of six) (Jones et al. 1993). The study by Bruins et al. (2003) reports 41% working part time.

Two studies report the percentage of people who were unable to work because of amputation. Kegel et al. (1978) found it to be 8% and Narang et al. (1984) only 3.5%. One quarter of employed amputees experienced periods of unemployment lasting more than 6 months since amputation (Millstein et al. 1985).

7.2.2 *Type of Work*

The percentage of people who returned to the same work also differs in various studies. It depended mainly on the type of work the people had done before amputation and the level of amputation. Narang et al. (1984) reported that only 12% of amputees returned to the same job. Over half of the people included in this study had been soldiers and had to change their profession as a result of amputation. In the USA, following amputation only 2.3% of soldiers remained on active duty, with 97% leaving the service (Kishbaugh et al. 1995). However, in some cases with good rehabilitation and appropriate prostheses they had been found to return to service, such as a return to active flying (Grossman et al. 2005). However, leaving the service did not mean that they were not working. Curley et al. (1982) report that 69% of amputee Vietnam Veterans were employed and Dougherty (1999) found that 70% of bilateral trans-femoral amputees from the Vietnam War were employed. Atesalp et al. (1999) reported that 31% of people after bilateral lower limb amputation because of landmine injury returned to the same job, but they did not provide details of the type of work they were employed to do.

Both veterans and civilians who had been engaged in physical labour before amputation have had to seek alternate jobs. The percentage of people who retain the same occupation following amputation ranges from 22 to 67% (Bruins et al. 2003; Fisher et al. 2003; Kegel et al. 1978; Millstein et al. 1985; Pedersen and Damholt 1994; Schoppen et al. 2001a). The lowest percentage is reported by Kegel et al. (1978), but only 60% of these people were of employable age. The highest has been reported by Schoppen et al. (2001a) who calculated it only for people working at the time of amputation. People who changed their occupation were more successfully reintegrated (90%) than those who did not change it (68%, Schoppen et al. 2001b). Only 58% of people with occupations that had a high physical workload returned to work. Some changed their jobs but stayed in the same workplace, others changed their workplace as well (Bruins et al. 2003; Fisher et al. 2003).

Most people who kept the same job following amputation had physically undemanding jobs (Bruins et al. 2003) and a lower level of amputation, mainly at the trans-tibial level (Kegel et al. 1978). Post-amputation jobs were generally more complex with a requirement for a higher level of general educational attainment and physically less demanding (Millstein et al. 1985; Pezzin et al. 2000; Schoppen et al. 2001a; Whyte and Carroll 2002). Whereas only 1% had been employed in a sedentary job prior to injury, 16% secured a sedentary job following amputation (Millstein et al. 1985), and only 21% returned to their pre-amputation job. Evaluations of how demanding the job was indicate a 30% decrease in the level of physical requirement compared to their previous job (Pezzin et al. 2000). The mean decrease in physical workload was 2.4 on a VAS scale (Schoppen et al. 2001b).

7.2.3 Time of Return to Work

The time taken to return to work following amputation is mentioned only in four studies (Bruins et al. 2003; Livingston et al. 1994; Rotter et al. 2006; Schoppen et al. 2001a). This ranges from 9 months for people after trans-tibial amputation (Bruins et al. 2003) to up to 2.3 years in the study by Schoppen et al. (2001a) for all people, independent of the amputation level. The most frequent reasons for delay were stump problems and problems in wound healing (85%), problems with the process of job reintegration (46%) and mental health problems (23%) (Bruins et al. 2003). Fifty-five percent of amputees stopped working in the first 2 years after amputation. Seventy-eight percent of them said that amputation-related factors played a role in their decision (Schoppen et al. 2001a).

7.2.4 Factors Influencing Return to Work

Factors influencing return to work can be divided into general factors, such as age, gender and educational level; factors related to impairments and disabilities because of amputation (Schoppen et al. 2001b); rehabilitation; prosthesis-related factors; and factors related to work and policies.

7.2.4.1 General Factors

Demographic factors such as sex and age at the time of amputation (Boynton 1955; MacKenzie et al. 2006; Nagarajan et al. 2003; Pedersen and Damholt 1994; Schoppen et al. 2001b; Schoppen et al. 2002; Whyte and Carroll 2002) and being white (Mackenzie et al. 2006; Pezzin et al. 2000) are found to have an effect on employment for people following amputation (Fisher et al. 2003; Millstein et al. 1985; Schoppen et al. 2001b). Whereas Millstein et al. (1985) reported women to have an unemployment rate 2.5 times greater than men, and older people as less successful in their return to work, Schoppen et al. (2001a) found fewer older men were employed but that age had no influence on the employment of women. Whyte and Carroll (2002) found a greater unemployment rate in women than in men. Teenagers with amputations as a result of bone tumours who were older than 12 years at the time of amputation (Nagarajan et al. 2003) and survivors of high-grade osteosarcoma (Yonemoto et al. 2007) were less likely to graduate from high school and college, compared to siblings.

The unemployment rate for amputees under 45 years was 22% compared to 48% for those over 45 years of age (Millstein et al. 1985). Only one out of five people who lost their job following amputation was younger than 45 years (Pedersen and Damholt 1994). People who were older at the time of amputation were more dissatisfied with reintegration into work activities (Nissen and Newman 1992).

People with lower educational level pre-injury had a lower reemployment rate and more of them had to change their jobs (Livingston et al. 1994; Nagarajan et al. 2003). Non-smokers and people with higher self-efficacy have a higher return to work (MacKenzie et al. 2006).

7.2.4.2 Factors Related to Impairments and Disabilities Due to Amputation

Factors related to impairments and disabilities because of amputation are: amputation level (Dougherty 1999; Hebert and Ashworth 2006; Jones et al. 1993; Livingston et al. 1994); multiple amputations (Whyte and Carroll 2002; Livingston et al. 1994); co-morbidity (Pezzin et al. 2000; Schoppen et al. 2001b); reason for amputation (Schoppen et al. 2001b); persistent stump problems (Livingston et al. 1994; Millstein et al. 1985); especially stump and phantom pain (Ide et al. 2002; Livingston et al. 1994; Millstein et al. 1985; Schoppen et al. 2001b; Whyte and Carroll 2002); the time from the injury to obtaining a permanent prosthesis (Livingston et al. 1994); physical comfort of the prosthesis (Schoppen et al. 2001b); and walking distance and restrictions in mobility (Fisher et al. 2003; Schoppen et al. 2001b). Twenty-eight percent of people with lower limb amputations experience problems finding work because of their amputation (Schoppen et al. 2001a).

Higher amputation levels decrease the reemployment rate. Jones et al. (1993), with a small sample, found two people working full time, one had trans-tibial amputation and the other trans-femoral. With a larger but still small sample Livingston et al. (1994) found no one with trans-femoral amputation returned to work, whereas 48% returned to work after trans-tibial amputation. Dougherty (1999) included only bilateral trans-femoral amputees from the Vietnam War. Sixteen (70%) were or had been employed outside the home even though the Veterans Administration provides adequate compensation to support their lifestyle (Dougherty 1999). Surprisingly Fisher et al. (2003) did not find the level of amputation and the cause of amputation correlating with the score on the employment questionnaire.

The reemployment rate was lower for people who sustained a work-related amputation (Livingston et al. 1994).

Studies that include pain have very different results. All of them include people after lower and upper limb amputation and do not distinguish between them when reporting the results. Millstein et al. (1985) found phantom and stump pain to be negatively associated with successful employment. Whyte and Carroll (2002) found that only phantom pain decreased employment, whereas Ide et al. (2002) found that the severity of all types of pain is not associated with return to work, but more severe pain decreases satisfaction with working life.

7.2.4.3 Rehabilitation

Livingston et al. (1994) found, with a small number of people, that inpatient rehabilitation had a negative influence on return to work. In their study, only 3 out of 14 patients who underwent inpatient rehabilitation returned to work in contrast to 14 out of 25 who were given outpatient therapy. The authors do not describe the criteria for the decision why someone underwent in- or outpatient rehabilitation, which might have influenced that result. With almost twice the number of people Pezzin et al. (2000) report that inpatient rehabilitation improved the health and vocational prospects of persons with trauma-related amputations. With calculations he assumed that additional ten nights of inpatient rehabilitation indicated a 14%age decrease in the number of people working fewer hours. Only 2 out of 33 patients were referred to vocational rehabilitation (Livingston et al. 1994). Vocational services have a positive effect on return to work (Millstein et al. 1985), but are not developed or do not form a part of rehabilitation programmes in all countries. For example, they are largely lacking in the UK (Fisher et al. 2003).

7.2.4.4 Prosthesis

To return to work people also need suitable and comfortable prostheses (Dasgupta et al. 1997; Grossman et al. 2005; Millstein et al. 1985), which may also prevent absence because of sickness and increase work efficiency (Dasgupta et al. 1997). People who frequently use prostheses are more likely to be employed (Millstein et al. 1985). Some also need additional adaptors and special components to be able to return to their previous work. For example, extra side rotator above the prosthetic knee enables pilots' entrance into the cockpit (Grossman et al. 2005).

7.2.4.5 Work and Policies Related Factors

Other factors that have been found to influence return to work are salary (Livingston et al. 1994), higher job involvement (MacKenzie et al. 2006), good support from the implementing body and the employer (Bruins et al. 2003; Boynton 1955;

Schoppen et al. 2001a) and social support networks (Boynton 1955; Livingston et al. 1994; Millstein et al. 1985).

Individuals who received social benefits and had a low pre-injury income in jobs which did not include medical benefits return to work less often (Livingston et al. 1994). When they have had a higher gross annual income more of them return to work (Hebert and Ashworth 2006). Almost one third report having fewer opportunities for job promotion (Schoppen et al. 2001a). In the study by Bruins et al. (2003) 34% had fewer promotion possibilities because of physical limitations and employers anticipating their going on sick leave in the future. Most patients who returned to work state that their current salary is less than that before their injury (Livingston et al. 1994; Millstein et al. 1985).

Forty-four percent report that job security is adversely affected by amputation (Millstein et al. 1985). Only a small number of amputees move up on the occupational classification scale, most move down by one to three levels (Whyte and Carroll 2002). Usually this results in a change from skilled to semi- or unskilled occupations (Whyte and Carroll 2002).

In Bruins et al. (2003) self-motivation was the essential factor for successful job reintegration, good support from the implementing body and the employer also being important. Insufficient support by the employer and the implementing body responsible for job reintegration were the most mentioned the most as obstacles to job reintegration (Bruins et al. 2003). Twenty-five percent of people did not experience any problems with work reintegration at all. Eight out of 14 people were dissatisfied with reintegration into work activities (Nissen and Newman 1992). Most of those people had amputation at the end of their careers; their average age at the time of amputation was 49 years (Nissen and Newman 1992).

Adjustments in the workplace are important for enabling persons to continue their work following amputation. Forty-three percent of people working before and following amputation mentioned modifications of their job as a factor in their ability to continue to work (Schoppen et al. 2001a). The adjustments are divided into four categories: changes in working time, getting aids (31%), changes in workload (31%) and other tasks or extra training (Schoppen et al. 2001a). When adjustments were necessary, most of the people took the initiative for them by themselves, they were seldom initiated by the rehabilitation team (Bruins et al. 2003). Twenty-seven percent of amputees said that they were partially dependent on others (Schoppen et al. 2001a) but reported that most colleagues and supervisors gave them sufficient consideration. People suitable for training on the job have a higher rate of return to work than those who require more extensive vocational preparation (Millstein et al. 1985).

Considering the increasing number of aged amputees, reduction of physical workload and adaptations in the workplace will be of extra important.

Seventy percent of working people judged their work life as good and 30% as unsatisfactory following amputation (Schoppen et al. 2002). Dissatisfied people had more comorbidities, lower mobility level and wished for more modifications in their workplace (Schoppen et al. 2002). The most important motives for returning to work were the value of their work as a way of spending the day and social contacts with colleagues and others (Bruins et al. 2003). Following amputation, most people believe that the most important factor for returning to work is their own attitude (Millstein et al. 1985).

7.3 Upper Limb Amputation and Work

7.3.1 Successful Return to Work

Employment rates of people following upper limb amputation are lower than employment rates for the general community (Davidson 2002). In Denmark the unemployment rate is twice that of the general population (Kejlaa 1992). Employment rate decreases even more if more elapses after the amputation (Davidson 2002).

It is also difficult to estimate the percentage of people with upper limb amputations who successfully return to work. In studies that include all people visiting a certain hospital or rehabilitation centre in a defined period of time it ranges from 53% (Kejlaa 1992) to 85% (Jones and Davidson 1995). There are great differences between studies conducted in different centres of the same country. Thus Jones and Davidson (1995) report an 85% re-employment rate for Royal South Sydney Hospital rehabilitation centre, whereas Davidson (2002) reports only 62% for New South Wales. The rate of employment or unemployment depends also on the definition selected and varies in one single study from 77.5 to 87.84% depending on the chosen definition (Millstein et al. 1985)

Studies that focus on a specific subgroup of people following upper limb amputation found the re-employment rate to be 100% for farmers (Reed 2004) and 61.3% for people amputated because of injury, who used body-powered prostheses (Stürup et al. 1988). The re-employment rate for people after finger or partial hand amputation ranges from 64% (Sagiv et al. 2002) to 72.2% (Burger et al. 2007).

There is no data on whether reemployed people worked full time and on the number of people who worked part time only.

7.3.2 Type of Work

Upper limb amputation has a significant impact on work. Whether a person following upper limb amputation will still be able to do the same work as before the amputation depends mainly on the type of work involved and the amputation level. Between 20 and 100% of people have to change their work after major upper limb amputation (Fernandez et al. 1993; Gaine et al. 1997; Hacking et al. 1997; Jones and Davidson 1995; Livingston et al. 1994; Wright et al. 1995).

Among the eight studies on partial hand amputation only Hattori et al. (2006) reported that all the people returned to the same job; however, he studied people following amputation of one finger only, with those of the thumb excluded.

Other studies report that people had to change their work in up to 47% of cases (Burger et al. 2007; Chow and Ng 1993; Lifchez et al. 2005; Sagiv et al. 2002). Musicians playing strings, keyboard or woodwinds have to change their job even if they have had an amputation of only the nail and nail bed (Dumontier 2003).

The greatest percentage of people, more than one half of all amputees, who have had to change their work following amputation are those who had unskilled manual work (Burger et al. 2007; Davidson 2002; Jones and Davidson 1995; Millstein et al. 1985; Sagiv et al. 2002), such as process workers, truck drivers, shop assistants or miners (Fernandez et al. 1993; Jones and Davidson 1995). Most of them changed their jobs to clerical work, services or went back to study (Davidson 2002; Jones and Davidson 1995; Millstein et al. 1985). While Fernandez et al. (1993) found that the lowest percentage of people returned to the agriculture sector, Reed (2004) reported that all farmers returned to their work very soon after major upper limb amputation. To explain these differences much better knowledge of social and work-related policies in different countries will be required.

7.3.3 Time to Return to Work

The amount of time it takes before people return to work following amputation ranges from 5 days to 24 months (Chow and Ng 1993; Livingston et al. 1994; Reed 2004). For people after finger amputation it is on average 4 months (Chow and Ng 1993) and is shorter than after finger replantation (Hattori et al. 2006). It is even shorter for most farmers who returned to work after 5 days to 6 months following a major upper limb amputation (Reed 2004). For them, depression is the main factor that delays return to work (Reed 2004). The amount of time it takes before people return to work may also depend on the cause of amputation. Patients after finger amputation due to work-related accidents may need longer time to return to work (7.5 months) than those who had other accidents (1.7 months) (Sagiv et al. 2002).

7.3.4 Factors Influencing Return to Work

7.3.4.1 General Factors

Return to work varies according to gender. Whereas Wright et al. (1995) and Millstein et al. (1985) found that women have a higher unemployment rate than men, Fernandez et al. (1993) found a greater proportion of retired and unemployed males. In evaluating this, we have to take into consideration that Millstein et al. (1985) did not distinguish between people with lower and upper limb amputation. Burger et al. (2007) found that more women than men were able to return to the same job as before amputation following partial hand amputation.

People younger than 50 years of age are more likely to return to-work than their older counterparts (Wright et al. 1995) and people older at the time of amputation are less successful in their return to work (Millstein et al. 1985) and more of them retire (Burger et al. 2007).

Education and years of education do not have a significant influence on keeping a job (Burger et al. 2007); however most people with lower levels of education have to change their job after amputation (Fernandez et al. 1993; Gaine et al. 1997; Hacking, et al. 1997; Jones and Davidson 1995; Livingston et al. 1994; Wright et al. 1995).

7.3.4.2 Factors Related to Impairments and Disabilities Due to Amputation

The lowest unemployment rate has been reported for people following trans-radial amputation (10%, Millstein et al. 1985; Stürup et al. 1988), although this has been higher in a more recent study (40%, Wright et al. 1995). The next lowest rate has been found for people with partial hand amputation (18%, Millstein et al. 1985) and trans-humeral amputation (22%, Millstein et al. 1985) although the latter has been found to be much higher in a later study (67%, Fernandez et al. 1993). People with amputation of three or more fingers are very seldom able to keep the same job after amputation (Burger et al. 2007). It seems that preservation of the elbow joint greatly improves working abilities.

Employment rate is also lower in people who have stump pain (Wright et al. 1995). All other studies include both: people following upper and lower limb amputation, and their conclusions are in the section above.

Dominance does not influence return to employment (Burger et al. 2007; Fernandez et al. 1993; Millstein et al. 1985) and has no influence on the type of work following amputation (Burger et al. 2007).

The only study reporting on how the *cause* of amputation may influence work found that few people who sustained work-related amputation returned to work (Livingston et al. 1994).

7.3.4.3 Rehabilitation

Only one study mentions factors related to rehabilitation. For return to work, time from amputation to the first fitting is important. If it is too long (longer than 12 weeks according to Gaine et al. 1997) people are less likely to work again.

7.3.4.4 Prosthesis

In spite of the great development in the field of upper limb prosthetics in recent years, we still do not have prostheses and components that resemble human hands. Usually decisions about prosthetic type and components depend on the type of work a person is doing, or will do, after amputation. Therefore studies that demonstrate high prosthetic use in employed persons and a positive correlation between the two (Burger et al. 2007; Davidson 2002; Millstein et al. 1985) may be interpreted as examples of where good clinical decisions have been made. But things are probably not so simple. There are some types of work for which prostheses are not as useful as for others or special components are needed. Some studies have also found that all non-users were employed (Stürup et al. 1988).

All unskilled persons were either occasional users or non-users of their body-powered prostheses (Jones and Davidson 1995). Most unskilled workers amputated owing to trauma used their body-powered prosthesis (Stürup et al. 1988).

Those whose occupation required sitting at a desk or supervising others appeared to use the myoelectric (Silcox et al. 1993) and silicone finger prosthesis (Burger et al. 2007; Hopper et al. 2000) more than those who performed manual labour. With new more durable myoelectric components that allow people also to work in wet and dusty conditions this may change. Over 80% of people use their myoelectric prosthesis for work (Pylatiuk et al. 2007).

7.3.4.5 Work and Policies-Related Factors

There are only a few studies about work factors and policy-related factors in samples comprised of people with upper limb amputations. The results are often in contradiction to each other.

Some find that the size of a company does not influence the return to work, whereas others conclude that it is a fundamental factor (Fernandez et al. 1993). In France, companies with 5,000 employees guarantee return to work (in the same post or a different one) whereas in small companies this return depends on the structure of the company itself, on the competence and initiative of the individual and on his ability to carry out another job (Fernandez et al. 1993).

By modifying the workstation and redesigning the task it is possible to make a job achievable or easier following amputation (Girdhar et al. 2001). Changes needed depend on the task, level of amputation and type of prosthesis (Girdhar et al. 2001).

The only study on the type of social security and work reports that social security is not a determining factor regarding return to work (Fernandez et al. 1993). More studies about these factors are needed to come to stronger conclusions.

7.4 Conclusion

Following amputation, people have several problems with returning to work. Many have to change their work and/or work only part time. Some also need modifications in their workplace. Their return to work depends on general factors, such as age at the time of amputation, sex and education, factors related to impairments and disabilities because of amputation and factors related to work and policies. Vocational rehabilitation and counselling should become a part of the rehabilitation programme after lower limb amputation for all people, who are at working age. Better co-operation between professionals, such as rehabilitation team members, implementing bodies, company doctors and the employers, is necessary.

For better understanding and stronger conclusions about the impact of different factors on the working abilities of people after amputation more well-conducted studies are needed.

References

Atesalp AS, Erler K, Gür E, Köse lu E, Kirdrmir V, Demiralp B (1999) Bilateral lower limb amputations as a result of landmine injuries. Prosthet Orthot Int 23:50–54

Boynton BL (1955) The rehabilitation and the re-employment potential of the amputee. Am J Surg 89:924–931

Bruins M, Geertzen JH, Groothoff JW, Schoppen T (2003) Vocational reintegration after a lower limb amputation, a qualitative study. Prosthet Orthot Int 27:4–10

Burger H, Marinček (2007) Return to work after lower limb amputation. Disabil Rehabil 29:1323–1329

Burger H, Maver T, Marinček (2007) Partial hand amputation and work. Disabil Rehabil 29:1317–1321

Chow SP, Ng C (1993) Hand function after digital amputation. J Hand Surg Br 18B:125–128

Curley MD, Walsh JM, Triplett RG (1982) Some adjustment indices of oral-maxillofacial war casualties, limb amputees, and noninjured veterans. Mil Med 147:572–574

Dasgupta AK, McCluskie PJA, Patel VS, Robins L (1997) The performance of the ICEROSS prostheses amongst transtibial amputees with a special reference to the workplace – a preliminary study. Occup Med 47:228–238

Davidson J (2002) A survey of the satisfaction of upper limb amputees with their prostheses, their lifestyle, and their abilities. J Hand Ther 15:62–70

Dougherty CP (1999) Long-term follow-up study of bilateral above-the-knee amputees from the Vietnam War. J Bone Joint Surg Am 81-A:1384–1390

Dumontier C (2003) Distal replantation, nail bed, nail problems in musicians. Hand Clin 19:259–272

Ebrahimzadeh MH, Rajabi MT (2007) Long-term outcomes of patients undergoing war-related amputations of the foot and ankle. J Foot Ankle Surg 46:429–433

Fernandez A, Revilla C, Su IT, Garcia M (1993) Social reintegration of juvenile amputees, comparison with a general population. Prosthet Orthot Int 27:11–16

Ferrapie AL, Brunel P, Besse W, Altermatt E, Bontoux L, Richard I (2003) Lower limb proximal amputation for a tumor, a retrospective study of 12 patients. Prosthet Orthot Int 27:179–185

Fisher K, Hanspal RS, Marks L (2003) Return to work after lower limb amputation. Int J Rehabil Res 26:51–56

Gaine WJ, Smart C, Bransby-Zachary M (1997) Upper limb traumatic amputees. J Hand Surg Br 22B:73–76

Girdhar A, Mital A, Kephart A, Young A (2001) Design guidelines for accommodating amputees in the workplace. J Occup Rehabil 11:99–118

Grossman A, Goldstein L, Heim M, Barenboim E, Dudkiewicz I (2005) Trans-femoral amputee pilots, criteria for return to the fighter cockpit. Aviat Space Environ Med 76:403–405

Hacking HGA, van der Berg JP, Dahmen KT, Post MWM (1997) Long-term outcomes of upper limb prosthetic use in the Netherlands. Eur J Phys Med Rehabil 7:179–181

Hattori Y, Doi K, Ikeda K, Estrella EP (2006) A retrospective study of functional outcomes after successful replantations versus amputation closure for single fingertip amputations. J Hand Surg Am 31A:811–818
Hebert JS, Ashworth NL (2006) Predictors of return to work following traumatic work-related lower extremity amputation. Disabil Rehabil 30:613–618
Hopper RA, Griffths S, Murray J, Manktelow RT (2000) Factors influencing use of digital prostheses in workers' compensation recipients. J Hand Surg Am 25A:80–85
Ide M, Obayashi T, Toyonaga T (2002) Association of pain with employment status and satisfaction among amputees in Japan. Arch Phys Med Rehabil 83:1394–1398
Jones LE, Davidson JH (1995) The long-term outcome of upper limb amputees treated at a rehabilitation centre in Sydney, Australia. Disabil Rehabil 17:437–442
Jones L, Hall LM, Schuld W (1993) Ability or disability? A study of the functional outcome of 65 consecutive lower limb amputees treated at the Royal South Sydney Hospital in 1988–1989. Disabil Rehabil 15:184–188
Kegel B, Carpenter ML, Burgess EM (1978) Functional capabilities of lower extremity amputees. Arch Phys Med Rehabil 59:109–120
Kejlaa GH (1992) The social and economic outcome after upper limb amputation. Prosthet Orthot Int 16:25–31
Kishbaugh D, Dillingham TR, Howard RS, Sinnott MW, Belandres PV (1995) Amputee solders and their return to active duty. Mil Med 160:82–84
Lifchez SD, Marchant-Hanson J, Matloub HS, Sanger JR, Dzwierzynski WW, Nguyen HH (2005) Functional improvement with digital prosthesis use after multiple digit amputations. J Hand Surg Am 30A:790–794
Livingston DH, Keenan D, Kim D, Elcavage J, Malagnoni MA (1994) Extent of disability following traumatic extremity amputation. J Trauma 37:495–499
MacKenzie EJ, Bosse MJ, Kellam JF, Pollak AN, Webb LX, Swiontkowski MF, Smith DG et al (2006) Early predictors of long-term work disability after major limb trauma. J Trauma 61:688–694
Mezghani-Masmoudi M, Guermazi M, Feki H, Ennaouai A, Dammak J, Elluch MH (2004) Facteurs lies à l'avenir fonctionnel et professionnel des amputés des members inférieurs appareillés. Ann Readapt Med Phys 47:114–118
Millstein S, Bain D, Hunter GA (1985) A review of employment patterns of industrial amputees – factors influencing rehabilitation. Prosthet Orthot Int 9(2):69–78
Nagarajan R, Neglia JP, Clohisy DR, Yasui Y, Greenberg M, Hudson M et al (2003) Education, employment, insurance, and marital status among 694 survivors of pediatric lower extremity bone tumors. Cancer 97:2554–2564
Narang IC, Mathur BP, Singh P, Jape VS (1984) Functional capabilities of lower limb amputees. Prosthet Orthot Int 8:43–51
Nissen SJ, Newman WP (1992) Factors influencing reintegration to normal living after amputation. Arch Phys Med Rehabil 73:548–551
Pedersen P, Damholt V (1994) Rehabilitation after amputation following lower – limb fracture. J Trauma 36:195–197
Pezzin LE, Dillingham TR, MacKenzie EJ (2000) Rehabilitation and the long-term outcomes of persons with trauma-related amputation. Arch Phys Med Rehabil 81:292–300
Pohjolainen T, Alaranta H, Karkkainen M (1990) Prosthetic use and functional and social outcome following major lower limb amputation. Prosthet Orthot Int 14:75–79
Pylatiuk C, Schulz S, Döderlein L (2007) Results of an internet survey of myoelectric prosthetic hand users. Prosthet Orthot Int 31:362–370
Reed D (2004) Understanding and meeting the needs of farmers with amputations. Orthop Nurs 23:397–405
Ross C, Mirowskay J (1995) Does employment affect health? J Health Soc Behav 36:230–243
Rotter K, Sanhueza R, Robles K, Godoy M (2006) A descriptive study of traumatic lower limb amputees from the hospital del Trabajador, Clinical evolution from the accident until rehabilitation discharge. Prosthet Orthot Int 30:81–86

Sagiv P, Shabat S, Mann M, Ashur H, Nyska M (2002) Rehabilitation process and functional results of patients with amputated fingers. Plast Reconstr Surg 110:497–503
Schoppen T, Boonstra A, Groothoff JW, de Vries J, Goeken LNH, Eisma WH (2001a) Employment status, job characteristics, and work-related health experience of people with a lower limb amputation in the Netherlands. Arch Phys Med Rehabil 82:239–245
Schoppen T, Boonstra A, Groothoff JW, van Sonderen E, Goeken LNH, Eisma WH (2001b) Factors related to successful job reintegration of people with a lower limb amputation. Arch Phys Med Rehabil 82:1425–1431
Schoppen T, Boonstra A, Groothoff JW, de Vries J, Goeken LNH, Eisma WH (2002) Job satisfaction and health experience of people with a lower-limb amputation in comparison with healthy colleagues. Arch Phys Med Rehabil 83:628–634
Silcox DH, Rooks MD, Vogel RR, Fleming LL (1993) Myoelectric prostheses. J Bone Joint Surg 75-A:1781–1789
Smith JJ, Agel D, Swiontkowski MF, Castillo R, Mackenzie E, Kellam JM (2005) Functional outcome of bilateral limb threatening – lower extremity injuries at two years postinjury. J Orthop Trauma 19:249–253
Somasundaram DJ, Renol KK (1998) The psychosocial effects of landmines in Cambodia. Med Confl Surviv 14:219–236
Stürup J, Tyregod HC, Jensen JS, Retpen JB, Boberg G, Rasmussen E, Jensen S (1988) Ttraumatic amputation of the upper limb, the use of body-powered prostheses and employment consequences. Prosthet Orthot Int 12:50–52
Whyte AS, Carroll LJ (2002) A preliminary examination of the relationship between emplyment, pain and disability in an amputee population. Disabil Rehabil 24:462–470
Wright TW, Hagen AD, Wood MB (1995) Prosthetic usage in major upper limb extremity amputations. J Hand Surg Am 20A:619–622
Yonemoto T, Ishii T, Takeuchi Y, Kimura K, Hagiwara Y, Tatezaki S (2007) Education and employment in long-term survivors of high-grade osteosarcoma, a Japanese single-center experience. Oncology 72:274–278

Chapter 8
Gender, Sexuality and Prosthesis Use: Implications for Rehabilitation

Craig Murray

Abstract One particular, highly personal, form of social relationship following amputation relates to sexual behaviour and related concerns. Although the role of relationships, and particularly romantic and sexual relationships, are generally important in most persons' lives, until relatively recently, the issue of sexuality following amputation has been a neglected area of research. This chapter summarizes the key literature on amputation and sexuality. This is mainly focused on males, who are lower-limb amputees, where data is collected via questionnaires or self-report surveys, with responses aggregated to ascertain the prevalence of certain pre-defined problems or issues. The sexual concerns of such persons can reasonably be expected to change over time and therefore to be different at various times following amputation and within the life course of individuals. Responses to limb losses are likely to be gendered experiences. Given the paucity of available literature on this topic and the importance of the issues surrounding it, this chapter reports the findings from a qualitative project of prosthesis use by both people with acquired amputations and those born with congenital limb deficiency on the complementary issues of gender, sexuality and romantic relationships. In this work, issues of sexuality emerged in relation to other salient meanings and experiences. In contrast to some prior research, which has had a tendency to explore sexual function and concerns in isolation, the qualitative analysis here highlights these as gendered concerns, and related to issues of forming romantic, and also sexual, relationships.

8.1 Introduction

This chapter is concerned with the gendered nature of prosthesis use, particularly as it relates to sexuality and the formation and maintenance of romantic relationships. Prior to presenting my own recent work on these interrelated topics, I begin with an overview of the current state of literature in this area.

C. Murray
School of Health and Medicine, Lancaster University, Lancaster, UK
e-mail: c.murray@lancaster.ac.uk

C. Murray (ed.), *Amputation, Prosthesis Use, and Phantom Limb Pain: An Interdisciplinary Perspective*, DOI 10.1007/978-0-387-87462-3_8,

A number of researchers have indicated that people with physical disabilities face difficulties in the formation and maintenance of sexual relationships (Taleporos 2001; Taleporos and McCabe 2001). Reasons for this include problems in sexual functioning (Whipple et al. 1996), individuals' confidence in establishing relationships (Taleporos and McCabe 2001), and a variety of environmental and social barriers to forming sexual relationships for people with physical disabilities, such as negative social attitudes, lack of privacy, reliance on other people for care and inaccessible homes and meeting places (Taleporos 2001; Taleporos and McCabe 2001).

A qualitative study conducted by Taleporos and McCabe (2001) identified a number of concerns that people with physical disability have in forming sexual relationships. Societal attitudes perceived people with physical disabilities as asexual and unattractive, which in turn limited or prevented them from establishing sexual partnerships. Such difficulties seem to exist for both men (Romeo et al. 1993; Shuttleworth 2000) and women (Rintala et al. 1997). Despite these problems, and although societal attitudes are frequently dismissive of the sexuality of persons with physical disabilities, they report the same desire and interest in physical touch, sexual intimacy and partnership as do the nondisabled (Edmonson 1988).

For people with physical disabilities in general, one particular, highly personal, form of social relationship following amputation relates to sexual behaviour and related concerns. The role of relationships, particularly romantic and sexual relationships, are generally important in most persons' lives. However, until relatively recently, the issue of sexuality following amputation was a neglected area of research (Goldberg 1984). A small collection of such studies has emerged over the last 25 years. This literature has largely focused upon sexual activities post amputation, either difficulties caused directly as a result of amputation such as loss of libido (Akesode and Iyang 1981), pain during sexual intercourse (Williamson and Walters 1996) or difficulties in sexual performance, such as adopting desired sexual positions as a result of the loss of a limb (Medhat et al. 1990).

In a recent systematic review of sexuality and amputation, Geertzen et al. (2009) found a number of issues discussed in the available literature. These include the observation that amputation had less of an impact on sexual functioning for married than single persons (Randall et al. 1945; Reinstein et al. 1978; Williamson and Walters 1996), older persons experienced a larger impact of amputation on sexual functioning than did younger persons (Bodenheimer et al. 2000; Williamson and Walters 1996) and those with phantom limb pain (PLP) and stump pain found a larger negative impact on sexual functioning than those who did not report such pain sensations (Akesode and Iyang 1981; Williamson and Walters 1996; Reinstein et al. 1978).

Geertzen et al (2009) found some variation between studies on how pervasive an issue or problem sexual functioning following amputation was, with one study reporting that this was not a serious problem (Bodenheimer et al. 2000), some studies with appreciable numbers of participants reporting some form of negative sexual functioning (Ide et al. 2002; Reinstein et al. 1978; Williamson and Walters 1996) and yet others with only a minority reporting definite problems (Akesode and Iyang 1981; Kejlaa 1992).

However, Geertzen et al. (2009) note that comparisons between these studies are hampered by the poor operational definitions of the outcome measures used, such as "sexual adjustment," "sexual functioning" or "sexual function." Moreover, because these studies tend to use cross-sectional designs, it is necessary to be cautious in making causal inferences about apparent associations. Geertzen et al. (2009) point out, for instance, the higher level of impact on sexual functioning in older persons with amputations might be an age-related effect unrelated to amputation.

Williamson and Walters (1996) found the majority (75%) of their participants reported restricting their sexual activities to some extent following amputation. Older age, not being married and greater feelings of self-consciousness regarding their amputation in intimate situations, were all predictive of less sexual activity. When amputation had a negative impact upon sexual activity, higher levels of depression were reported.

In a more recent survey of males with lower-limb amputations, Bodenheimer et al. (2000) sought to describe their sexual and psychosocial functioning. Although the participants' level of interest in sex was high (90% of the sample), many experienced orgasmic (63%) and erectile (67%) problems. However, Williamson and Walters (1996) note that research has shown that with a supportive spouse or partner, higher levels of sexual activity among amputees are reported. The overall contribution of sexual satisfaction to quality of life has been investigated by Walters and Williamson (1998), where the degree of satisfaction reported by amputees with their sexual relationships was found to predict overall quality of life. The results were discussed in terms of implications for interventions aimed at improving adjustment to limb amputation.

Although the work reported in these studies provide valuable insights into the importance of sexual functioning following amputation, the manner by which such issues are experienced and addressed remain under explored, particularly with regards to the formation and maintenance of romantic relationships. For example, in a comparison of the quality of life in bone tumor patients who had either had a lower-limb amputation or a limb salvage operation, Postma et al. (1992) found that among the single patients, 65% of those with amputations reported difficulty in developing relations with the opposite sex, whereas only one of the limb-salvage patients did so, echoing the difficulties reported in the literature for persons with physical disabilities in general. Also 65% of those with amputations felt embarrassed to show their prosthesis and restricted themselves from certain social activities, whereas none of the limb salvage patients did so. Work such as this is suggestive of the need for further research to examine how relationships with members of the opposite sex are encountered and managed following limb loss and prosthesis use.

Although the body of available literature on sexuality issues for people following amputation is small, there has been even less consideration of such issues pertaining to people born with congenital limb deficiencies, where either the absence or deformity of an anatomical limb or limb part necessitates the use of an artificial limb. One notable exception is the work of Gelya Frank. Frank (1984) provides a life history of Diane DeVries, a woman born without legs and with above-elbow stumps, in which she emphasises the normalcy of her participant's body for her. In this paper Frank emphasises themes of "cultural normalcy" and "orientation to independent living"; these themes convey the normal cultural development of Diane's life in relation to her age, gender and social background, which includes initiation into sex, falling in love and living with a partner.

Frank's work with Diane DeVries is an illustrative example of the potential of such qualitative work to examine how amputation or limb absence is experienced in the context of the formation and maintenance of sexual and romantic relationships. Frank provides a detailed qualitative analysis of such experiences, but although the qualitative approach taken by Frank provides a rich understanding of her participant's experiences, this is limited due to its focus on one woman with congenital limb deficiency. The experiences and meanings for both males and females, whether they have acquired limb loss or congenital limb deficiency, remain overlooked. However, understanding of such experiences can reasonably be expected to aid a variety of health professionals involved in the rehabilitation of this client group to address these sensitive topics, which are often difficult for the patient to raise.

Williamson and Walters (1996) found patients express relief and appreciation when professionals affirm their sexuality (Williamson and Walters 1996), and Badeau (1995) notes they are often interested in finding out how various aspects of their rehabilitation, such as medication, will impact on their libido. However, research demonstrates that medical practitioners are often reluctant to discuss sexual intimacy with disabled patients (Lewis 1990), so that issues of sexuality are often left unaddressed during rehabilitation (Schover and Jensen 1988), often in part because of the adoption of negative societal attitudes which view people with physical disabilities as asexual or unable to attract a partner.

The available literature on amputation and sexuality is mainly focused on male, lower-limb amputees, where data is collected via questionnaires or self-report surveys, with responses aggregated to ascertain the prevalence of certain pre-defined problems or issues. However, although the sexual concerns of such persons can reasonably be expected to change over time, and therefore to be different at various times following amputation and within the life course of individuals, and responses to limb loss are likely to be gendered experiences, these very issues have not been researched to date.

An alternative to the quantitative, structured approaches to data collection and analysis which is available on these topics is qualitative work in which the views and experiences of persons with amputations are sought, so that the findings are grounded in the issues which participants themselves identify as being of importance.

To begin to redress the paucity of available literature on this topic and to address the importance of the issues surrounding it, the present chapter presents the findings from a study of prosthesis use by both people with acquired amputations and those born with congenital limb deficiency on the complementary issues of gender, sexuality and romantic relationships.

8.2 A Qualitative Exploration of Gender, Sexuality and Prosthesis Use: Study Background

The analysis presented in the present study is drawn from a wider project, conducted over a 2 year period, examining the feeling and experience of prosthesis use (Murray 2004, 2005, 2009). The research took a multi-method qualitative approach, with research data being drawn from semi-structured interviews conducted face-to-face and via electronic mail, as well as from electronically stored communication between conversants on two publicly available computer forums over a 2-year period. The participants were 16 males and 19 females. Twenty-seven of these had limb loss; 24 of these were of the lower limb and three were of the upper-limb. Eight participants had congenital limb absence; four of these were of the lower limb and four were of the upper-limb. The age range for the whole of the sample was 16–75. In addition, posts to two electronic discussion groups over a 2 year period were analyzed.

A list of topics provided a provisional structure to the interview. This included (where appropriate) questions regarding participants' responses to amputation, any concerns they had about the future, the immediate impact of amputation upon their life, feelings about using prostheses, the importance of cosmetic appearance, and changes to disablement as a result of prosthesis use. The schedule did not include any specific questions regarding the issues of gender, romantic relationships, sexuality or sexual concerns. Rather, these were either first offered by participants in discussions in response to other questions asked during the interviews, or were observed in the discussions which took place in the on-line discussion groups. The primary data were analysed using Interpretative Phenomenological Analysis (IPA) (Smith 2004). This particular form of qualitative analysis was selected because of its emphasis on both the life world of participants, and how this occurs and is made sense of in social interaction. IPA is an approach intended to explore how participants experience their world, and hence enables an insider's perspective of the topic under study. The process of analysis derives themes from the data itself, rather than analysing data on the basis of pre-defined categories.

8.2.1 Data Examples of Gendered Concerns, Sexuality, Romantic Relationships and Prosthesis Use

It is important to note, as indicated earlier, that the interview schedule did not include any specific questions regarding the issues of gender, romantic relationships, sexuality or sexual concerns. The way in which such concerns are volunteered and expressed by participants therefore becomes an important consideration in judging the degree to which the research findings here reflect and are grounded in participants, personal feelings, as opposed to being dictated by the concerns or interests of the researcher. Whereas some of the issues arising from the present work have been discussed in depth elsewhere (Murray 2005, 2009), here attention is given to two interrelated themes, namely: *The prosthesis and gendered identities*; and *Barriers and facilitators to forming romantic and sexual relationships.*

Issues of sexuality emerged in relation to other salient feelings and experiences. In contrast to some prior research, which has had a tendency to explore sexual concerns in isolation, the qualitative analysis here highlights these as gendered concerns, and related to issues of forming romantic and sexual relationships. The analysis which follows therefore begins with a discussion of gendered concerns, before moving on to presenting issues surrounding romantic and sexual relationships.

8.2.1.1 The Prosthesis and Gendered Identities

For male participants, the issue of gender and prosthesis use came up in discussions of gendered roles. These were often what could be described as normative, traditional or stereotypical characterisations of the male gender role, such as the family "breadwinner" and in descriptions of strength. Here prosthesis use was important in allowing men to continue providing financially for their family, and prostheses were valued for allowing or enabling strenuous activities. Such views are evident in, and typified by, the following interview extract:

> For me it was important that I could get back to work and sort the finances of the family. My wife had taken on a job that she had had before our son was born, and I wanted to have things back to normal as soon as possible. The [prosthetic] leg allowed me to do this, and I was soon back repairing the house (back on ladders), and putting in 12 h per day of physically demanding work. [Steve, aged 54, right above knee amputation 14 years previously. Email interview]

While masculinity was implicated in prosthesis use, as described above, for female participants in particular, the gendered nature of prosthesis use was of personal significance. Here, participants often spoke of the frustration they had encountered in obtaining prosthetic limbs that were appropriately gendered. In fact, for some female prosthesis users, artificial limbs that had been provided to them were designed for male users. The affront to a person's sense of femininity on such occasions had profound personal significance;

> I probably would not have retained some anger at a prosthetist who put men's feet on my limbs _if_he_had_told_me_ that only men's feet were available at any point in time! [Post made to on-line discussion group]

However, for some female participants, a prosthetic designed for use by males was sometimes more appropriate for their needs. As the following interview excerpt demonstrates, the prosthetic that had been designed for use by females was too small for the participant, who then had to use an alternative which was originally designed for a male;

> Participant: This is a man's hand. I used to have really long nails and everything before hand, but you can't really have long nails with that.

Interviewer: Why have you got a man's hand?

Participant: Because the ladies hand, I looked at it and said "it's a tiddly that." It is, it's too small. I mean, I've always done quite hefty work in my jobs, so I suppose it's given me quite muscular type hands. And this to me was more like my hand than what the other tiddly things were, you know. [Val, aged 52, left, below elbow amputation 51/2 years previously. Face-to-face interview]

Some females perceived prosthesis use, particularly upper-limb prostheses, as not suitable for females. A lack of cosmesis and the view that women have "more of a problem" with wearing prostheses were cited as reasons for non-use:

I know that having another [prosthetic] arm would make life much easier in many respects, but my reason for not using them has been largely cosmetic. It seems that women have more of a problem with wearing a hook than men (blame it on Peter Pan, if you will!) and I admit, I am one of them. [Karen, 25 years old, right above knee amputation 2 years previously. Email interview]

The design of a prosthetic could create problems for gendered identities, but, even when prostheses were appropriately female-gendered, participants often found that they were designed for a much older female. As such, a person's self-identity as a prosthetic user could then be placed within an older age group:

It took me several years to learn how to get a good fit. I didn't know the difference between a prosthetist and a prosthetic technician. I went to one firm where the prosthetist was also an orthopedic surgeon; the client saw him once, and only saw the technicians thereafter, for years. These technicians decided to give me a light duty SACH foot appropriate for a 60 year old female, despite my telling him that I walked several miles each day. The foot broke while I was walking from their firm back to my dorm! [Post made to on-line discussion group]

Clothes emerged as important in females' sense of femininity. Where prosthesis use compromised what could be worn, particularly those items most traditionally worn by females, participants expressed their disappointment:

And even now, like, I've got some lovely suits, but with being short, only five foot, I cannot have a heel – the heel I'm wearing, my limbs are all made for that heel. So I cannot go into high heels. So, I can never wear a nice two-piece, and I'd love to have been able to do that. [May, aged 73, left, below knee amputation 62 years previously. Face-to-face interview]

These issues highlight the importance of gendered identities in prosthesis use which have been missed or overlooked in other, more structured, quantitative work that has looked at sexual functioning following amputation. So, for example, research which has attempted to address the issue of gender, amputation and prosthesis use has had mixed findings. Kasharni et al. (1983) found women were more likely than men to be depressed following an amputation. However, a larger body of research has found that gender does not predict levels of psychosocial adjustment (Bradway et al. 1984; Dunn 1996; Rybarczyk et al. 1992). However, it is clear from participants in the project discussed here that gender, and more specifically femininity, is highly implicated in females' experience of prosthesis use. This becomes further apparent later, when considering issues of romantic and sexual relationships.

8.2.1.2 Barriers and Facilitators to Forming Romantic and Sexual Relationships

A concern with romantic and sexual relationships, prior and post amputation, and related to prosthesis use was evident in the research interviews and in the messages of the email discussion groups. This was a theme which was echoed, although with different emphases, by both males and females, particularly those who were single or in short-term relationships at the time of amputation, and therefore may be related to the findings of research which shows that single individuals experience more difficulties post-amputation than do married persons (Parkes 1975; Randall et al. 1945). The following excerpt is that of a male recalling his feeling on this issue soon after his own amputation:

> [There was] the nagging awful thought that while I am essentially the same person I was before the wreck, I also had a leg missing and this might really repulse any woman I might be interested in getting to know. This was of *great* concern to me. [William, aged 54, right below knee amputation 27 years previously. Email interview]

The feeling that amputation was a change which presented a challenge to the acceptability and desirability of the person was compelling for male participants. As such, relationships of relatively short duration which were in place at the time of amputation were considered to be not what their partner had "signed on" for, and in some cases led to a desire to seek out new partners, in part to prove that they could be willingly rather than grudgingly accepted as they were, with their limb loss;

> As a man, my prospective may be a bit different. But one of my biggest problems when I first had to deal with my amputation was the feeling that I would not be able to find a girlfriend. This is a bit odd, as I was engaged at the time, but I felt like she did not sign on to be with an amputee, and that she should not have to stay with me.... I was feeling sorry for myself, and kind of wanted to prove I could find someone who would like me, even if I was an amputee. [Post made to on-line discussion group]

The concealment and revealing of prosthesis use was discussed by participants in relation to romantic relationships and encounters. For some prosthesis users an artificial limb was considered as highly visible and a hindrance to the formation and maintenance of romantic relationships. The following participant, a young female who had lost her arm in an accident 1 year previously, evaluated her limited use of her prosthesis almost exclusively in terms of attractiveness and dating:

> I will use a prosthetic for practical reasons, if there is no way I can manage without one, but I don't feel it's something I will use all day, every day, or something that will become a part of me or my identity. What it seems to boil down to is that the prostheses I have now are clumsy, look really unattractive and take so much effort to learn how to use them effectively that I don't think it warrants going through the psychological trauma of getting used to people staring at me wherever I go. Call me vain, but I can't imagine myself going on a "hot date" brandishing my prosthesis with a hook (let alone a clamp) on the end! [Karen]

Women with physical disabilities have been found to be less satisfied with their dating frequency than able bodied women, and to perceive more constraints in attracting partners, along with more societal and personal barriers to their dating (Rintala et al. 1997). Such concerns in the work reported here were sometimes dramatically bolstered by others' actions. The following excerpt is from a new subscriber to an on-line discussion group, who describes her rejection by her boyfriend post-amputation as being "dumped like a broken Barbie Doll," and shows her own concern for the likelihood and viability of future romantic relationships:

> I am a recent amputee (traumatic, above the knee). This is all new to me. I am interested in e-mail with experienced amputees. Right now I am having a lot of trouble with pain in my leg, the one that is no more. Before the accident I was very active, what can I still do? Last, for now, my boyfriend dumped me like a broken Barbie Doll, what are my chances of finding a guy that will accept my new body? [Post made to on-line discussion group]

Related to the above, we can consider Young's (1990) phenomenology of female body experience, in which she argues that the "typical" contradiction of female embodiment is the tension between the female subject as embodied agent and the female body as object. This is a problem of the lived body, and the objectified body. Because of this, female self-identity, particular in young females, may rest to a large extent upon their sense of physical attractiveness. The example provided above might reasonably be expected to happen to a new male amputee; however, in over 2 years of on-line discussions, as well as interviews, men were not found to describe being rejected by a partner because of their amputation.

The below post to an online discussion group highlights the complexity surrounding the interrelated issues of physical contact and desire for a sexual relationship:

> Hello I am new here and I have been an amputee for almost 4 years now.... I have been having bad feelings as though no one will accept me and that I will never be loved. I know my son loves me but that's different. I crave physical intimacy and not only that but I want to be married. I just feel like whenever I go out in public that people will not want to engage in conversation or be bothered with me because of my disability. My son's father helps out but he doesn't understand me totally. I just want to be accepted by other people and hopefully meet someone who will love me for me. Is there anyone who can help with what I am going through? [...] even while with my son's father, I just did not feel comfortable touching him because I thought it made him feel funny. I never spoke with him about this because it is embarrassing to me but now I have stopped all relations with him since thanksgiving. I want to be with him but don't feel sexy nor attractive. He doesn't say anything about the amputation but states that he doesn't know me any other way. We have had some fights and he says he is done with me but I want us to make it work for our son. I will be counseling soon in hopes that I can learn to be more outgoing and approachable. I want to be able to desire sex again as well as attain new relationships. [Post made to on-line discussion group]

Williamson and Walters (1996) noted that amputation-related changes in physical self-esteem and perceptions often led to feelings of being undesirable and could be related to aspects of sexual functioning. The above post demonstrates how amputation may have long-lasting impact on perceptions of attractiveness, even when relationships are formed post-amputation. Lack of libido does not indicate lack of interest in sexual activity, as the above participant relates how she "craves" physical contact and hopes to "desire" sex once more. Moreover, sexual and romantic relationships are not seen in isolation from other social relationships but, rather, being liked, loved, or sexually desirable all share a common concern with acceptance and belonging.

In relation to these issues, Shakespeare (1996) notes that people who become disabled in adulthood are often faced with psychosexual consequences that can be among the most difficult results of traumatic injury. Disabled men are more likely than women to maintain their relationships following a disability, with women often being left by their partner (Shakespeare 1996). The availability of a supportive spouse or an equivalent partner has repeatedly been shown to predict higher levels of sexual activity among amputees (Postma et al. 1992). Walters and Williamson (1998) found that satisfaction with one's sexual relationships with others predicted overall quality of life in a sample of adult amputees, although a general decrease in sexual activity by people with an amputation has been reported (Williamson and Walters 1996). However, being in a relationship, even in one formed after amputation, may still be characterised by concerns regarding sexual desirability and sexual interest, as shown here.

While sexual issues were clearly of importance to research participants, not everyone had worries concerning the formation of romantic and or sexual relationships. Rather, for some participants what was important was their ability to participate in the social rituals which circumscribed courtship rituals. This can be illustrated by the following comments made by one female interviewee, Rachel, regarding the use of her prosthetic hand. Rachel discussed how her prosthetic integrated her into an important social ritual of adolescent courtship. However, what is important here is not that the prosthetic facilitated romantic or sexual relationships – indeed the respondent remarks she "usually had three boyfriends at a time" – but, rather that it enabled participation in a social ritual, one in which the conventional use of the body was of central importance.

> The reason I wanted it [the prosthetic] when I was sixteen – remember I was a teenager, very popular, I usually had three boyfriends at a time [laughs]. "Sweet sixteen and never been kissed," I'd been kissing boys since I was thirteen. To me kissing was absolutely lovely. I always had lots of boyfriends. But when I was dancing it was nice to have a hand to put on their shoulders. It was a cosmetic reason really, but I was pleased to have it. [Rachel, 65 years old, right, below elbow, congenital limb deficiency. Face-to-face interview]

The comments of this participant therefore indicate the central role of a prosthesis in aiding courtship rituals, which may underpin the maintenance of romantic relationships and are missed by quantitative research designs which assess overall level of satisfaction with sexual or social relationships.

In this research, in general, upper-limb prostheses were thought to be more visible. Lower limb prostheses were more likely to be viewed as "concealed." While previous work has shown how this invisibility might be of value, for example in getting yourself across as a person before choosing if and when to disclose amputation and prosthesis use (Murray 2005), this hidden aspect of limb loss/absence and prosthesis use itself was often a source of anxiety in courtship rituals, as evidenced in the below female participant's comments:

> When I was weary, you know when you first start going out with your girl friends, that was, I can remember going into clubs, you know where they have turns on the stage and, you know, a club. But not like now [laughs]. And, erm, a doorman at the door. And I used to be

sat there with a friend, Irene. We'd see these boys coming towards us and I'd think please god don't let him ask me to dance. But it doesn't bother everybody. I've seen loads of young girls, they're very very confident at the centre. You know. But I hated it. And then me mum tells, she says "don't you realise that, they don't [know about the amputation and prosthesis use], you're making them embarrassed. Those poor young men, they don't know, they just think you're being awful." I used to say "oh I don't dance." And they'd say, "well you can just shuffle around on the floor." And it was awful. And that's what I didn't like. But, I got over it. [Sarah, aged 54, left, below knee amputation 42 years previously. Face-to-face interview]

8.3 Discussion

Within this chapter I have overviewed the key literature relating to gender, sexuality, romantic relationships and prosthesis use before presenting relevant data on these issues from a large scale qualitative project.

With the exception of one early study that found that women experienced depression more frequently than men following an amputation (Kasharni et al. 1983), gender has generally not been found to predict levels of psychosocial adjustment (Bradway et al. 1984). However, previous research has overlooked the gendered context of prosthesis use, and how this might impact upon the experiences of prosthesis users. The present work begins to addresses this research gap, and demonstrates that gender is an important aspect of prosthetic identity. In the case of males, gender roles, such as the male "breadwinner" were highlighted. Here prosthesis use was important in allowing men to continue providing financially for their family, and prostheses were valued for allowing or enabling strenuous activities.

However, the gendered nature of prosthesis use was generally more pronounced for female participants. Some respondents had been provided with prosthetic limbs that were designed for, and looked like, men's limbs. On such occasions the participants' sense of femininity could be undermined. For females, the ability to wear items of clothing that can be seen as quintessentially "feminine" was important for their sense of self-identity. Clothes worn prior to limb loss and prosthesis use, such as high heels, were therefore often still worn, even when this made prosthesis use more difficult and threatened the participants' health. Moreover, participants often found that even when their prosthetic had been designed for a female, they were often designed for a much older female. As such, a person's self-identity as a prosthetic user could then be placed within an older age group.

This differs from the use of clothing as discussed by Kaiser et al. (1985, 1987) in the management of appearance by persons with physical disabilities. Whereas Kaiser's research found that disabled persons attempted to appear as normative as possible through their clothing choices, using a variety of techniques to conceal or deflect attention away from their disabilities (as did some of my own participants), here participants often wanted to wear clothes that were important for their sense of identity, but did not necessarily make it any easier to conceal a prosthetic.

A number of participants reported a great deal of anxiety regarding their sense of sexuality and sexual attractiveness. As Kelly (1992) argues, both sexuality and sexual relationships are the core of social life, with people's self-perception often strongly linked with their capacity to engage in sexual relationships. Kelly (1992) found in his research with ileostomy patients that sexual relationships became a difficult precinct of their lives. While the person with an ileostomy appears and acts "normally," the very private area of sexual relationships reveals in a vivid manner the deviant nature of their body. Sexual relations are one strong example of a wider problem in social interaction for people with disabilities. In this research, these problems and difficulties associated with general self-presentation and impression management were much discussed but were particularly sensitive with regard to actual or potential romantic and sexual encounters.

The findings presented here add support to earlier recommendations to facilitate discussion about sexuality in the rehabilitation process to help address patients' sexuality-based anxieties which, in turn, can help to improve their quality of life (Walters and Williamson 1998). The work presented here highlights the importance of both sexual and romantic relationships in the overall quality of life for amputees. In addition, it explicates the various ways in which meaning is given to sexual relations, and how new (and old) relationships are (re)formed and (re)built upon the background of limb loss/absence and prosthesis use. There is still a need for further research to identify the specific dimensions of sexuality that increase satisfaction, facilitate rehabilitation, and contribute to the quality of life as called for by Williamson and Walters (1996) some time ago, and for which they recommended qualitative methodologies to assess the differential construction of sexuality post amputation that they saw as necessary for successful interventions. The present research, which examined the spontaneous accounts offered by participants on these issues, is one small step towards this call.

References

Akesode FA, Iyang UE (1981) Some social and sexual problems experienced by Nigerians with limb amputation. Trop Geogr Med 33:71–74

Badeau D (1995) Illness, disability, and aging. Sex Disabil 13:219–237

Bodenheimer C, Kerrigan AJ, Garber SL, Monga TN (2000) Sexuality in persons with lower extremity amputations. Disabil Rehabil 22:409–415

Bradway JK, Malone JM, Racy J, Leal JM, Pool J (1984) Psychological adaptation to amputation: An overview. Orthot Prosthet 38(3):46–50

Dunn DS (1996) Well-being following amputation: Salutary effects of positive meaning, optimism and control. Rehabil Psychol 41(4):285–302

Edmonson B (1988) Disability and sexual adjustment. In: Van Hasselt VB, Strain PS, Hersen M (eds) Handbook of development and physical disabilities. Pergamon Press, New York, pp 91–106

Frank G (1984) Life history model of adaptation to disability: The case of a "congenital amputee". Soc Sci Med 19(6):639–645

Geertzen JHB, Van Es CG, Dijkstra PU (2009) Sexuality and amputation: A systematic literature review. Disabil Rehabil 31(7):522–527

Goldberg RT (1984) New trends in the rehabilitation of lower extremity amputees. Rehabil Lit 45:2–11
Ide M, Watanabe T, Toyonage T (2002) Sexuality in persons with limb amputation. Prosthet Orthot 26:189–194
Kaiser SB, Freeman CM, Wingate SB (1985) Stigmata and negotiated outcomes: Management of appearance by persons with physical disabilities. Deviant Behav 6(2):205–224
Kaiser SB, Wingate SB, Freeman CM, Chandler JL (1987) Acceptance of physical disability and attitudes toward personal appearance. Rehabil Psychol 32(1):51–58
Kasharni JH, Frank RG, Kasharni SR, Wonderlich SA (1983) Depression among amputees. J Clin Psychiatry 44:256–258
Kejlaa GH (1992) The social and economic outcome of upper limb amputation. Prosthet Orthot Int 16:25–31
Kelly M (1992) Self, identity and radical surgery. Sociol Health Illn 14(3):390–415
Lewis CE (1990) Sexual practices: Are physicians addressing the issues? J Gen Intern Med 5:S78–S81
Medhat A, Huber PM, Medhat MA (1990) Factors that influence the level of activities in persons with lower limb amputation. Rehabil Nurs 15:13–18
Murray CD (2004) An interpretative phenomenological analysis of the embodiment of artificial limbs. Disabil Rehabil 26(16):963–973
Murray CD (2005) The social meanings of prosthesis use. J Health Psychol 10(3):425–441
Murray CD (2009) The personal meanings of prosthesis use. Disabil Rehabil 31(7):573–581
Parkes CM (1975) Psychosocial transitions: Comparison between reaction to loss of a limb and loss of a spouse. Br J Psychiatry 127:204–210
Postma A, Kingma A, DeRuiter JH, Koops HS, Veth RPH, Goeken LNH, Kamps WA (1992) Quality of life in bone tumor patients comparing limb salvage and amputation of the lower extremity. Journal of Surgical Oncology 51:47–51
Randall GC, Ewalt JR, Blair H (1945) Psychiatric reaction to amputation. J Am Med Assoc 128:645–652
Reinstein L, Ashley J, Miller KH (1978) Sexual adjustment after lower extremity amputation. Arch Phys Med Rehabil 59:501–504
Rintala DH, Howland DC, Nosek MA, Bennett JL, Young ME, Foley CC, Rossi CD, Chanpong G (1997) Dating issues for women with physical disabilities. Sex Disabil 15:219–242
Romeo AJ, Wanlass R, Arenass S (1993) A profile of psychosexual functioning in men following spinal cord injury. Sex Disabil 11:269–276
Schover LR, Jensen SB (1988) Sexual problems in chronic illness: A comprehensive approach. Guilford, New York
Shakespeare T (1996) Power and prejudice: Issues of gender, sexuality and disability. In: Barton L (ed) Disability and society: Emerging issues and insights. Longman, London, pp 191–214
Shuttleworth R (2000) The search for sexual intimacy for men with cerebral palsy. Sex Disabil 18:263–282
Smith JA (2004) Reflections on the development of interpretative phenomenological analysis and its contribution to qualitative research in psychology. Qual Res Psychol 1(1):39–54
Taleporos G (2001) Sexuality and physical disability. In: Wood C (ed) Sexual positions: An Australian view. Hill of Content Publishing, Melbourne, pp 155–166
Taleporos G, McCabe MP (2001) Physical disability and sexual esteem. Sex Disabil 19:131–148
Walters AS, Williamson GM (1998) Sexual satisfaction predicts quality of life: A study of adult amputees. Sexuality and Disability 16(2):103–115
Whipple B, Richard E, Tepper M, Komisaruk B (1996) Sexual response in women with complete spinal cord injury. Sex Disabil 14:191–201
Williamson GM, Walters AS (1996) Perceived impact of limb amputation on sexual activity: A study of adult amputees. J Sex Res 33:221–230
Young I (1990) Throwing like a girl and other essays in feminist philosophy and social theory. Indiana University Press, Indiana

Chapter 9
Post Amputation Chronic Pain Profile and Management

Jai Kulkarni and Kate Grady

Abstract The pain profile following amputation is complex and can be considered as an amalgam of acute post-operative pain, nociceptive pain of the stump, neuropathic pain of the stump, phantom limb pain, mechanical back pain, and pain in more remote sites (such as proximal ipsilateral joints, the contralateral limb) caused indirectly by amputation of the limb. The composition of the pain profile is variable with often more than one of the above co-existing although not all pains necessarily being present and is temporally dependent, varying at different stages of the peri-operative and post operative period. Such complexity makes pain after amputation difficult to manage. Each component of the overall pain experience should be identified and addressed separately.

9.1 Introduction

The causation of lower limb amputations in the United Kingdom has changed in the last 70 years, subsequent to the Second World War, from trauma to dysvascularity as the main factor. Dysvascularity related to peripheral vascular disease and diabetes is now noted to be the most common cause of lower limb amputations in the UK.

Data from the 2005–2006 National Amputee Statistical Database Group (NASDAB 2005) indicates that dysvascularity is the cause of lower limb amputation in 75% of presentations. By rough estimates there are approximately 50,000 lower limb amputees in the United Kingdom and recent NASDAB data indicates that 5,000 amputees were referred to various Disablement Services Centres for amputee/prosthetic rehabilitation in 2005/2006. Of these, 50% were over the age of 65 and 25% were over the age of 75. The median age for males was noted to be 65 years, for females 69 years.

Lower-limb amputations account for 91% of amputee referrals, with 5% being for upper limb amputations, and 4% in the congenital/other causative factors group.

J. Kulkarni (✉)
Department of Rehabilitation Medicine, DSC University Hospitals of South Manchester, M20 1LB, UK
e-mail: jai.kulkarni@uhsm.nhs.uk

C. Murray (ed.), *Amputation, Prosthesis Use, and Phantom Limb Pain: An Interdisciplinary Perspective*, DOI 10.1007/978-0-387-87462-3_9,

An amputee becomes "established" 1 year post-amputation. At this stage pain that resolves spontaneously will have done so and the remaining pain can be considered a steady state situation requiring detailed assessment and expert management. However, residual stump pain, phantom pain and in particular the mechanical pains can develop many years after amputation. Sufferers of post amputation pain should be referred early to a specialist clinic. As with all ongoing pain problems a full bio psycho-social assessment should be made and attention and treatment given to any associated behavioural, maladaptation, mood disorder or disorder of cognition needs. Co-existing depression should be treated and cognitive behavioural therapy contemplated. (Smith et al. 1999).

9.1.1 Acute Post-Operative Pain

This is a normal phenomenon. There should be an awareness of the potential for acute post-operative neuropathic pain and where this is identified by pain being associated with sensory disturbance and descriptors such as "shooting", "stabbing", "burning", "cramping" it should be treated early.

9.1.2 Nociceptive Pain in the Stump

One-third of the amputees have nociceptive stump pain. This is usually related to the following:

1. Abnormal stump tissues: There can be "give" of the myoplasty in the amputated stump with consequent prominence of the distal end of the bone in the stump.
2. Adherent scars.
3. Localised infection, folliculitis or epidermoid cysts.
4. Allergic phenomena due to prosthetic materials, stump liners, stump socks or application of local creams for donning or doffing of the sockets of the artificial limb prostheses (Lyon et al. 2000).
5. Ill fitting sockets of the artificial limb prosthesis.
6. Stump claudication, particularly in dysvascular patients with or without diabetes and for those for whom an ischaemic cause precipitated amputation.
7. Painful jactitation (jumping movements).

9.1.3 Neuropathic Pain of the Stump

Neuropathic pain occurs when an insult to a nerve causes changes in the peripheral and central nervous system. It is strongly correlated to phantom pain; it has been found to be present in 61% of those with phantom pain and only in 39% of those without phantom pain (Sherman and Sherman 1983; Sherman and Arena 1992).

Neuropathic pain is identified by its descriptors. Words such as sharp, burning, cramping and stabbing are used or adaptation of such fierce sensations such as of boiling oil on the stump. There may be a background pain, or paroxysmal pain only or background pain and paroxysms may co-exist. There can be associated sensory abnormalities such as hyperathia (pain in an area of numbness), allodynia (a painful response to a normally non-painful stimulus) and hyperalgesia (a heightened pain response to a painful stimulus).

Neuropathic pain can be non-specific and due to generalised involvement of the nerves or following amputation surgery neuromata can develop where cut nerves attempt to re-grow forming bulbous ends, and sprouting collaterally. Nerves are normally embedded by surgical technique away from the incision line. The neuroma is pressure sensitive and is a source of excruciating pain if it is tethered and in a direct weight bearing area. Troublesome neuromata should be diagnosed by MR scan, and where found surgical excision is an option. However, in the absence of pathology it is advised that stump revision surgery is avoided.

9.1.4 Phantom Limb Pain

The presence of phantom limb sensation is noted to be in almost 100% of the cases, often with sensations of distortion of shape, length and position (e.g. leg can feel bent under them or as if going through the bed) and telescoping (where the distal portion of the phantom feels nearer to the stump than it would be in an intact limb). Phantom sensations tend to diminish over time. Phantom sensation and phantom pain are strongly correlated. It has been shown that phantom pain was present in 36 out of 37 amputees with phantom sensations but only in 1 out of 17 without phantom sensation (Kooijmann et al. 2000)

Estimations of the frequency of phantom limb pain vary from 10% to 100%. Eighty-five percentage of our patient population complain of an element of phantom limb pain which is in keeping with other studies (Grady and Kulkarni 2001).

Phantom limb pain is more likely to occur in adults than children. If phantom pain does not occur in the few days or weeks after amputation it is less likely to occur in these patients than in those in whom it presents in the early post-operative period. The incidence of phantom pain has been reported at 92.3% at 1 week, and 78.8% at 6 months. It can be delayed in onset beyond the time of the amputation and may first occur after trauma (even of a relatively minor nature) to the stump or stump revision surgery.

Phantom pain is intermittent, demonstrates neuropathic features such as gripping, burning, squeezing, drilling and can be more intense in the distal part of the phantom such as fingers/hand, toes/feet as these are better represented on the sensory homunculus.

Uncontrolled pre-amputation pain is a risk factor for the development of phantom pain. However, results from studies which have attempted to reduce the incidence of phantom pain by various methods of controlling pre-amputation pain have produced inconsistent results. Further phantom pain can mimic uncontrolled pre-amputation pain in both character and site.

It is recognised that psychological distress, anxiety and depression can accompany any chronic pain syndrome and no more so than in phantom pain because of the associated losses and reminders of the loss.

9.2 Treatment and Management

In principle treatments should be aimed at the specific cause and non-pharmacological treatments are preferable to drug treatments.

9.2.1 Acute Post-Operative Pain

This is treated and managed conventionally by non-steroidal, opioids and regional local anaesthetic techniques.

9.2.2 Management of Nociceptive Stump Pain

Good stump hygiene and stump sock care is essential to avoid sweat maceration and infection. Recurrent folliculitus can be obviated to some extent by depilation with local hair removal creams and/or laser depilation.

We advocate routine use of Hibiscrub stump washes, followed by use of Dermol 500 soaps and in specific cases local antibiotic, Fucidin ointment. If there is a fungal element likely to be present, then use of Daktacort cream can be of benefit. In most cases sweat rashes settle on their own or with cautious use of 1% hydrocortisone cream. Friction related local problems can be obviated by siliconised liners. Epidermoid cysts are common in the flexural hair areas and may eventually need surgical intervention.

Pain related to ill-fitting prostheses is treated by refitting of the sockets and using newer materials which are silicone based liners, flexible sockets and compatible interfaces. Treatment of stump claudication, starts with assessment of flow by Doppler studies and may warrant vascular surgical referral. A give of stump myoplasty may need combined assessment with the plastic surgeon and surgical intervention. We advocate the concept of combined clinics between involving the rehabilitation specialist and the plastic surgeon and the rehabilitation specialist and the pain management specialist.

9.2.3 *Management of Neuropathic Stump Pain and Phantom Pain*

9.2.3.1 Non-Pharmacological Interventions

1. Movement, massage and manipulation of the stump in a gentle regular manner can be of assistance in desensitising where there is hypersensitivity.
2. Transcutaneous nerve stimulation has been shown to give relief.
3. Biofeedback can be helpful in burning and cramping phantom pain.
4. Relaxation therapy and hypnotherapy can be of assistance.
5. By observing the reflection of the normal limb in a mirror in the position of the phantom allows some patients to be able to generate voluntary movements of relaxation in the phantom limb to relieve the pain of clenched fingers or toes.
6. Acupuncture/electro acupuncture can lead to some alleviation of pain.
7. Immersive Virtual Reality treatment approach can give releif.

9.2.3.2 Pharmacological Treatment

Pharmacological treatment of both neuropathic pain of the stump and phantom pain is based on the treatments used for other neuropathic pain conditions. Tricyclic antidepressants, some anticonvulsants, opioids and lignocaine plasters are the mainstay of treatment for neuropathic pain.

9.2.3.3 Antidepressants

Amitriptyline is most commonly used, although Nortriptyline has a less sedating effect and may therefore be preferred. A starting dose of 10 mg every night in the elderly and 25 mg in younger patients is recommended. As side affects allow, the dose can be increased by small increments at weekly intervals. Patients should be told that minor side effects decrease with time, and that they should avoid alcohol and attention should be given to fitness to drive. The analgesic effects of the Tricyclic antidepressants have been shown to be independent of their effect on mood. It is important that this is explained to patients.

The antidepressant drugs, which act by serotonin/noradrenaline uptake inhibition such as Venlafaxine are sometimes used in the management of neuropathic pain.

9.2.3.4 Anticonvulsants

Gabapentin does not have significant drug interactions and has a favourable safety profile though dizziness and sedation is common. Our own audit studies have indicated that Gabapentin is most efficacious at a dose of 900–1,800 mg daily.

Some patients use it on an as need be basis. The dose recommendations are to reach a range of 900–1,200 mg daily, by dose increments of 100 mg. Gabapentin can be used in combination with a tricyclic antidepressant (Grady and Kulkarni 2002).

Pregablin can certainly be of benefit for this group of patients. We tend to start at a lower dose of 25 mg and build the dose up to either 75 mg twice a day or 150 mg twice a day. Lamotrigine is effective in some neuropathic pains but can require doses of up to 600 mg leading to some adverse skin reactions and some impairment in vision. Dose titration needs to be taken cautiously. Sodium Valporate and Phenytoin are less commonly used as compared to Gabapentin/Pregablin. Clonazepam can be tried at a doses of 0/5–1.5 mg every night particularly if there is an element of agitation or sleeplessness.

9.2.3.5 Other Drugs

Mexilitine and other memory stabilising drugs have been used for neuropathic stump and phantom pain. Intravenous Ketamine has been shown to produce some reduction in phantom and stump pain. Beta blockers have been reported as effective in the relief of phantom limb pain. Calcitonin injections have been used in some studies. Tizanidine hydrochloride is an alpha adrenergic agonist, which is used in increased tone and spasticity has been used in the treatment of stump jactitation – jumping in the stump which can trigger pain.

9.2.3.6 Local Creams

Capsaicin is a cream available for treatment of post-hepatic neuralgia, painful diabetic neuropathy and osteoarthritis of the knees but is reported to be useful in treating neuropathic pain of the stump. It needs to be applied cautiously on a 4 times a day basis. The therapeutic effect can be delayed up to 6 weeks into treatment and hence needs a fair amount of persistence on behalf of the patient. It may cause localised burning sensation which can be exacerbated by perspiration inside the stump sock. This may be attenuated by application of Lignocaine gel 10 min before the cream. The burning sensations usually cease after 3 weeks when the Lignocaine can be stopped. Lignocaine 5% patches assist in very local stump pain. Strontium compound creams may have some effect in local stump pain.

9.2.3.7 Injection Treatments

Pain related to lower limb amputation which is sympathetically maintained maybe decreased by injection of local anaesthetic to the lumbar sympathetic plexus. This can be effective and the duration of effect tends to outlast the normal pharmacological duration of the local anaesthetic. Pain can be triggered by defaecation, micturition or sexual intercourse and this would suggest it is a sympathetically maintained pain which can be manipulated by epidural local anaesthetic injections. In cases where dysvascularity contributes to pain the post chemical sympathectomy effect of vasodilatation can be therapeutic. Occasional local stump injections of lignocaine/bupivacaine into trigger spots of tender areas or superficial neuromas can be used.

9.2.3.8 Neurostimulation

Transcutaneous nerve stimulation with a TENS machine and also use of electro acupuncture can be of assistance. In some recalcitrant cases assessment and usage of Spinal Cord Stimulator or deep brain stimulator can be considered. Careful selection of these patients is very important.

9.2.3.9 Low Back Pain

Unilateral major lower limb amputation results in lifelong disturbance of biomechanics even with good prosthetic rehabilitation. Frequency of mechanical back pain increases, our own published study has indicated that this back pain is mainly due to disturbed biomechanics rather than degenerative changes (Kulkarni et al. 2005). Management of back pain is a multidisciplinary one with emphasis on attention to alignment and length of the prosthesis and emphasis on mobility and rehabilitation.

9.2.3.10 Proximal Joint Arthritis Related Pain

Lower limb amputees have an increased frequency of arthritis in the contralateral and ipsilateral proximal joint. Our peer review publication indicated that the frequency can be 3–6 times more than the normal cohort. Careful attention to socket fit and alignment can lead to improvement in gait pattern and decrease in abnormal forces from the proximal and contralateral joints (Kulkarni et al. 1998).

Attention also needs to be focussed on the customised suspension element of the prosthesis. In some cases local treatment of intra-articulator hydrocortisone and local anaesthetic may be of assistance; with the recalcitrant patient, one needs to address the issues pertaining to joint replacement/arthroplasty.

9.3 Conclusion

Hence, overall in our opinion, these patients with chronic post-amputation pain are best served by a combined consultant clinical review with the rehabilitation specialist and the pain specialist and in particular cases, where surgical intervention is necessitated, involvement of the plastic surgery team. A structured approach as outlined above is recommended in chronic post amputation pain management.

References

Grady K, Kulkarni J (2001) How to relieve chronic pain after amputation. Pulse Clin 61(18):72–75

Grady K, Kulkarni J (2002) Effectiveness of Gabapentin for control of phantom limb pain – open label prospective study. Pain Soc Newsl 1(17):4–5

Kooijmann CM, Dijkstra PJ, Teertzen JHB et al (2000) Phantom pain and phantom sensations in upper limb amputees: an epidemiological study. Pain 87:33–41

Kulkarni J, Adams J, Thomas E, Silman A (1998) Association between amputation, arthritis and Osteopenia in British male war veterans with major lower limb amputations. Clin Rehabil 12(4):354–361

Kulkarni J, Gain W, Buckley J, Rankine J, Adams J (2005) Chronic low back pain in traumatic lower limb amputees. Clin Rehabil 19:81–86

Lyon CC, Kulkarni J, Zimerson E, Van Ross E, Beck MH (2000) Skin disorders in amputees. J Am Acad Dermatol 42:501–507

National Amputee Statistical Database (NASDAB) (2005) Crown Copyright. Edinburg. UK. www.nasdab.co.uk

Sherman RA, Arena JAG (1992) phantom limb pain: mechanisms, incidence and treatment. Crit Rev Phys Rehab Med IV(1–2):1–26

Sherman R, Sherman C (1983) Prevalence and characteristics of chronic phantom limb pain among American veterans: results of a trial survey. Am J Phys Med 62:227–238

Smith DG, Ehde DM, Legro MW, Ariberge D, Boone DA (1999) Phantom limb pain, residual pain and back pain after lower extremity amputations. Clin Orthop 361:29–38

Chapter 10
Phantom Limb Pain; Prevalence, Mechanisms and Associated Factors

Cliff Richardson

Abstract This chapter reviews the literature regarding phantom limb pain (PLP) following limb amputation. Controversies exist over the incidence and prevalence, causes, mechanisms and management of PLP. Owing to a lack of effective treatment for the condition, interest has turned to the potential to pre-empt PLP. Pre-emption needs targets, and interest has focused upon pre-amputation pain. A lack of success with pain pre-emption has led to interest in other factors which may be associated with PLP. To ensure rigour, before addressing factors that are associated with PLP, it is necessary to tackle controversies within PLP. Each area of controversy will be reviewed with the final section concentrating on those aspects, inherent within an individual, that play a role in PLP development and/or maintenance.

10.1 Background

It is widely accepted that the French military surgeon Ambrose Pare was the first to report phantom phenomena following amputation, in the mid-sixteenth century (Harwood et al. 1992; Lyth 1995; Weinstein and Anderson 1994; Wesolowski and Lema 1993; Weinstein 1998). Pare wrote of his incredulity when amputee soldiers stated that they were still aware of the missing limb. Disbelief was the established medical view that led Silas Weir Mitchell to publish the first detailed study of the phenomenon in a general, rather than a medical journal, in the nineteenth century. It was within Weir Mitchell's study that the term "phantom" was coined for the first time (Weir Mitchell 1871).

Since Weir Mitchell's work, phantoms have been reported following the removal of virtually every body part including teeth, tongue, breast, bladder, anus and genitalia (Battrum and Gutmann 1996; Biley 2001; Dijkstra et al. 2007; Hanowell and Kennedy 1979; Fainsinger et al. 2000; Fisher 1999) and have been reported in people with paraplegias and when a limb is congenitally absent (Melzack and Loeser 1978; Melzack et al. 1997; Wilkins et al. 2004).

C. Richardson (✉)
Adult Nursing, University of Manchester, Manchester, UK
e-mail: clifford.richardson@manchester.ac.uk

C. Murray (ed.), *Amputation, Prosthesis Use, and Phantom Limb Pain: An Interdisciplinary Perspective*, DOI 10.1007/978-0-387-87462-3_10,

All of these conditions involve deafferentation. Deafferentation occurs when the peripheral nerve supply is disconnected from the central nervous system. The body part that has been deafferented can, but does not always, develop into a phantom. The relationship between deafferentation and phantoms has led to an increase in research activity investigating the neuronal pathways and neurochemical nature of nerves following deafferentation as there are variations between individuals. Differences in sensations including the presence of pain in phantom body parts have been reported. As phantom limbs have been the most researched, the rest of the chapter will concentrate on these.

10.1.1 Phantom Phenomena in Amputated Limbs

A phantom has been defined as "the continuous awareness of a (or part of a) non-existing or deafferented body part with specific form, weight, or range of motion" (Ribbers et al. 1989). Most amputees report that they have an awareness of the limb (phantom), and some report this awareness in terms of exteroceptive descriptors such as "pins and needles" or "itch" (Montoya et al. 1997). Early papers proposed that increased exteroceptive amplitude could explain phantom limb pain (PLP), but this remains unproven. Other amputees describe an embodiment without sensation (Hunter et al. 2003; Richardson et al. 2006). They know the phantom is there but have no feeling in it. Irrespective of whether sensation is present, the phantom embodiment is always perceived innately by the amputee (Melzack 1992).

Kinetic (movement) and kinaesthetic (positional orientation) sensations are also widely reported. The phantom may move spontaneously (often referred to as spasm which can be painful) or remain fixed, while some amputees are able to move the phantom at will. Kinaesthetically, a phantom can take up any position in space and should not be assumed to take up a natural position in relation to the contra-lateral limb (*see* Figure 10.1). There have been reports that phantoms can be held outstretched in front, behind or sideways.

Telescoping is a commonly reported form of kinaesthesia. Here the phantom shortens (usually over time), so that in extreme cases, only the digits remain on the end of or within the residual limb (stump). There has been a belief that PLP reduces as telescoping occurs; however, two studies have challenged this principle by being unable to establish a link between the two phenomena (Montoya et al. 1997; Richardson et al. 2006).

Stump pain (SP) is a recognised chronic pain associated with amputation with an approximate 50% prevalence (Richardson et al. 2006). Its aetiology remains unclear, but there are clear associations between SP and PLP.

Super-added sensations, a collection of different types of sensation, have also been reported. Most of these are non-painful feelings that the limb is clothed or that a watch is present on the phantom wrist (Katz and Melzack 1990; Wesolowski and Lema 1993); however, there have been some reports that previous pains such as old in-growing toenails can also be felt (Katz 1992; Melzack 1992).

Only two studies have quantified super-added sensations. The first identified 5 of 68 (7%) amputees (Katz and Melzack 1990), and the second found that 8 out

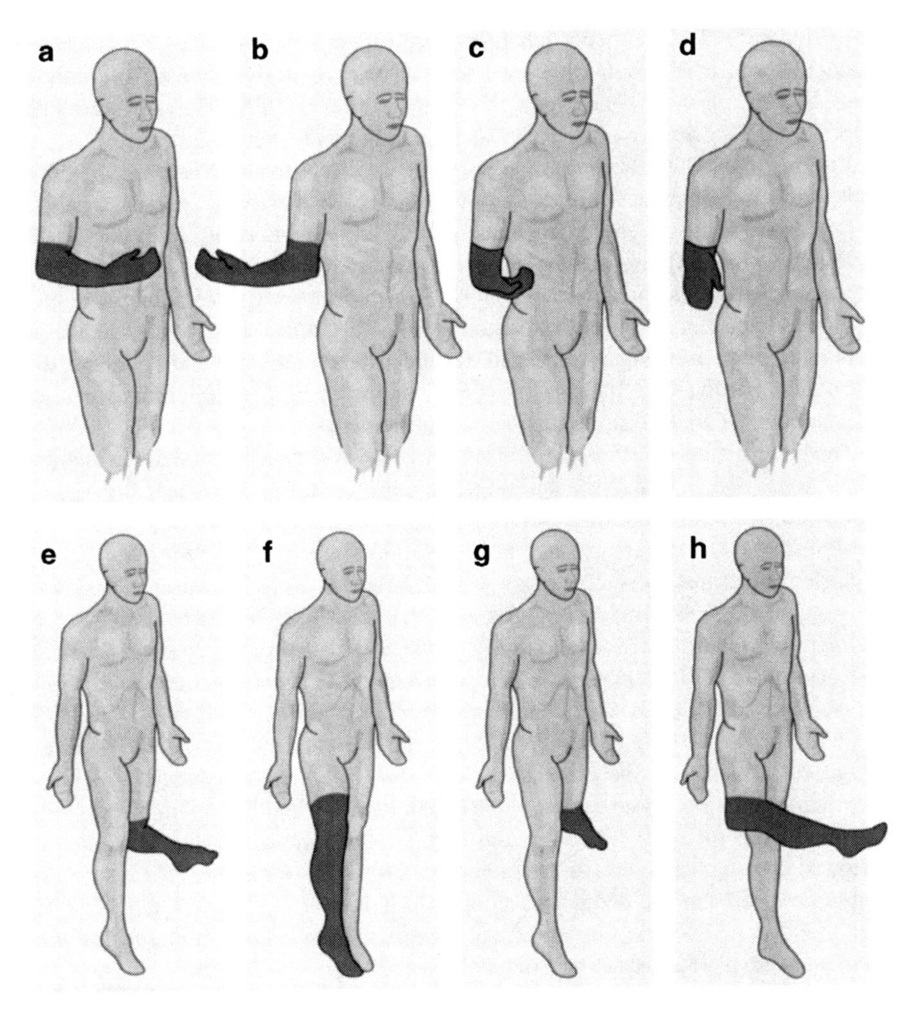

Fig. 10.1 Kinaesthetic seusations for limb amputees (a-d upper limb; e-h lower limb) (Shadow areas = phantom)

of 52 (15.4%) lower limb amputees reported that their phantom was clothed (Richardson et al. 2006). As discussed later, these sensations suggest that a neuronal memory system may be active to generate or maintain the phantom.

10.1.2 Phantom Limb Pain

PLP is defined as "Painful sensations referred to the absent limb" (Nikolajsen and Jensen 2000). The initial incredulity of Ambrose Pare and generalised medical scepticism led to the denial of PLP, predisposing a common assumption that it was psychogenic in origin (Finnoff 2001; Jensen and Nikolajsen 2000; Patterson 1994;

Rounseville 1992). This belief has taken into account all amputees, but has been especially true in children and those who were born limb deficient (McMahon 1998; Melzack et al. 1997; Weinstein 1998; Wilkins et al. 1998). However, research over the last 20 years supports PLP as a real and organic pain.

PLP prevalence has been reported as 2–88% by Jensen and Nikolajsen (1999). Systematic variations in study methodologies and samples have been cited as the main reason for the difference in these figures (Smith et al. 1999); however, a lack of clarity in the definition of the sensations reported by amputees is likely to be important (Kalauokalani and Loeser 1999). Most of the early studies did not define or discuss the different sensations, and it is easy to postulate that the prevalence of PLP could be over or under estimated dependent upon attitudes and beliefs of the researchers involved. It could be possible, for instance, to misinterpret phantom sensations or SP as PLP if they are not distinguished.

The better organised studies of the last 15 years have endeavoured to make these distinctions, and in doing so, the range of prevalence has narrowed. Prevalence figures between 50% and 67% have been reported in varying samples (upper and lower limb) and by different methods (survey and interview) across many different countries (Kooijman et al. 2000; Davis 1993; Jensen et al. 1983; Jensen et al. 1985; Montoya et al. 1997; Pohjolainen 1991; Smith et al. 1999; Wartan et al. 1997).

Even higher levels were found in a retrospective cross-sectional survey study of 255 amputees (56% response rate) in which the PLP prevalence level was 72% (Ehde et al. 2000). Other studies that had found prevalence levels as high as 79% tended to be the better organised and larger sample sized studies (Houghton et al. 1994; McCartney et al. 1999; Sherman et al. 1984) The same percentage (78%) was also identified in a more recent prospective study wherein 59 amputees were recruited prior to lower limb amputation due to peripheral vascular disease and followed up 6-months later (Richardson et al. 2006). The strength of this last study comes from having a homogenous group of amputees. The highest rate (79.6%) was found in 437 lower limb amputees identified from a limb-fitting centre who were on average 18.8 years since amputation (Dijkstra et al. 2002).

In summary, it can be concluded that the prevalence of PLP is somewhere between 50% and 80%, but as the studies with larger sample sizes have tended to give higher prevalence, it is likely that the true figure is at the top end of that range. In Britain during the year 2005/6, there were 5,835 major limb amputations and a further 4,425 hand and foot amputations (DOH 2008); hence PLP will affect a substantial number of new people each year, and there is a need to learn more about the condition so that the sufferers can be managed.

10.1.2.1 Description and Intensity of PLP

PLP has been described as tingling, uncomfortable, pins and needles, throbbing, sharp, stabbing (knifelike), burning, squeezing, jabbing, like an electrical current, cramping, crushing, itching, tearing, shooting and has often been described as being similar to pain experienced prior to amputation (Knox et al. 1995; Krane and Heller 1995; Lyth 1995; Sherman et al. 1992; Williamson 1992; Wilkins et al. 1998; Yetser 1996).

Overall intensity of PLP on a 10 cm visual analogue scale (VAS) has ranged from 2.7 to 7.7 (Houghton et al. 1994; Richardson et al. 2006; Sherman et al. 1984; Wartan et al. 1997).

10.1.2.2 Temporal Elements of PLP

PLP has two forms, background and exacerbations. Both aspects vary over time; for instance the number of exacerbations and length of each exacerbation show considerable fluctuation. This variation can be measured in different ways including the length and number of exacerbations per day and the number of days per week exacerbations are experienced. Background PLP also fluctuates.

10.1.2.3 Mechanism for PLP

A widely agreed and accepted mechanism for PLP does not yet exist. Initially, interest focused upon the peripheral nerves, but inconsistencies between individuals led to a widening of the search for answers. Any proposed mechanism has to pull together evidence from the periphery, the spinal cord and the brain including the cortex. Various mechanisms have been proposed including cortical reorganisation and pain memory; however, there are missing elements within each of these. A single overarching theory explaining all the physical and psychological attributes and individual variations is required. The neuromatrix theory proposed by Melzack in 1992 could be such a theory (Melzack 1992). The neuromatrix theory will be discussed after all the contributing physiological evidence has been reviewed.

10.1.2.3.1 Peripheral Nerve Involvement

Following amputation, the excised nerves can form irritable foci and neuromata. It is assumed that as these nerves originally served areas distal to the stump, any impulses from the excised nerve will "automatically" be interpreted centrally as arising from the now missing limb (Harwood et al. 1992; Herbener 1988; Melzack 1992; Nikolajsen and Jensen 2001; Ribbers et al. 1989; Weinstein and Anderson 1994).

If this were the mechanism for PLP, it would be expected that excision of neuromata, irritable foci and/or the introduction of local anaesthetics would control PLP. This has not, however, been a very successful method of treatment (Herbener 1988; Hill 1999; Stannard 1993). Scrutiny has turned to the neural connections along the pain pathways away from the stump (Coderre and Katz 1997), making the spinal cord the next area of study.

10.1.2.3.2 Evidence of Spinal Cord Involvement

Impulses enter the spinal cord via the dorsal horn, creating a cascade. This cascade leads to the transmission of impulses via varying pathways up the spinal cord and into the brain. The synaptic interchange within the dorsal horn can be altered depending on the input from the periphery and from the brain. Following nerve injury such as deafferentation after amputation, changes occur in the dorsal horn, including disinhibition, the depletion of Substance P and the modification of the levels of endorphins. This is a different response to those seen when normal noxious stimuli are received, and it has been proposed that these changes represent a potential mechanism for PLP (Hill 1999; Nikolajsen and Jensen 2000; Ribbers et al. 1989; Rounseville 1992; Stannard 1993; Weinstein 1998; Wesolowski and Lema 1993). It is a powerful argument; however, as these changes seem to be ubiquitous after deafferentation, they do not give the reason why some individuals do not experience PLP after amputation. Focus has therefore turned to the brain and higher centres.

10.1.2.3.3 The Brain/Higher Centres

Following deafferentation, neural processing changes have been seen in various areas of the brain (Harwood et al. 1992; Stannard 1993; Williams and Deaton 1997). Evidence of neural plasticity and cortical reorganisation has been forthcoming following improvements in imaging techniques with the sensory areas becoming the most implicated in the development of PLP. The Penfield map of the sensory cortex is shown in (*see* Figure 10.2).

In an imaginative experiment in upper limb amputees, an American group identified that the use of touch, pinprick and warmth to the face of upper limb amputees would often produce phantom sensation in the missing hand. By moving the stimuli across the ipsilateral lip and cheek, a total map of the hand was produced (Ramachandran and Rogers-Ramachandran 1996; Ramachandran et al. 1992). A second map of the hand was also found on the stump. Inspection of the sensory homunculus in the cortex shows the hand is flanked on one side by the face and the other by the upper arm (*see* Figure 10.2); hence the suggestion is that following amputation, the areas of the cortex that used to respond to sensory information in the hand, are taken over by the areas adjacent to them. This has been termed cortical reorganisation or cortical re-mapping.

Following these early findings, a significant positive linear relationship ($p=0.0001$) between PLP and cortical reorganisation was identified (Flor et al. 1995). Indeed amputees without PLP showed minimal capacity to re-map onto the face or stump. The same group went further by testing 8 male upper limb amputees with PLP and/or phantom sensations and comparing them to a group of 8 healthy non-amputee controls (Knecht et al. 1996). They confirmed that cortical reorganisation has to occur for PLP to exist.

Interestingly, studies designed to visually portray the return of the limb using specialised prostheses or mirror boxes have shown that PLP can be reduced and that

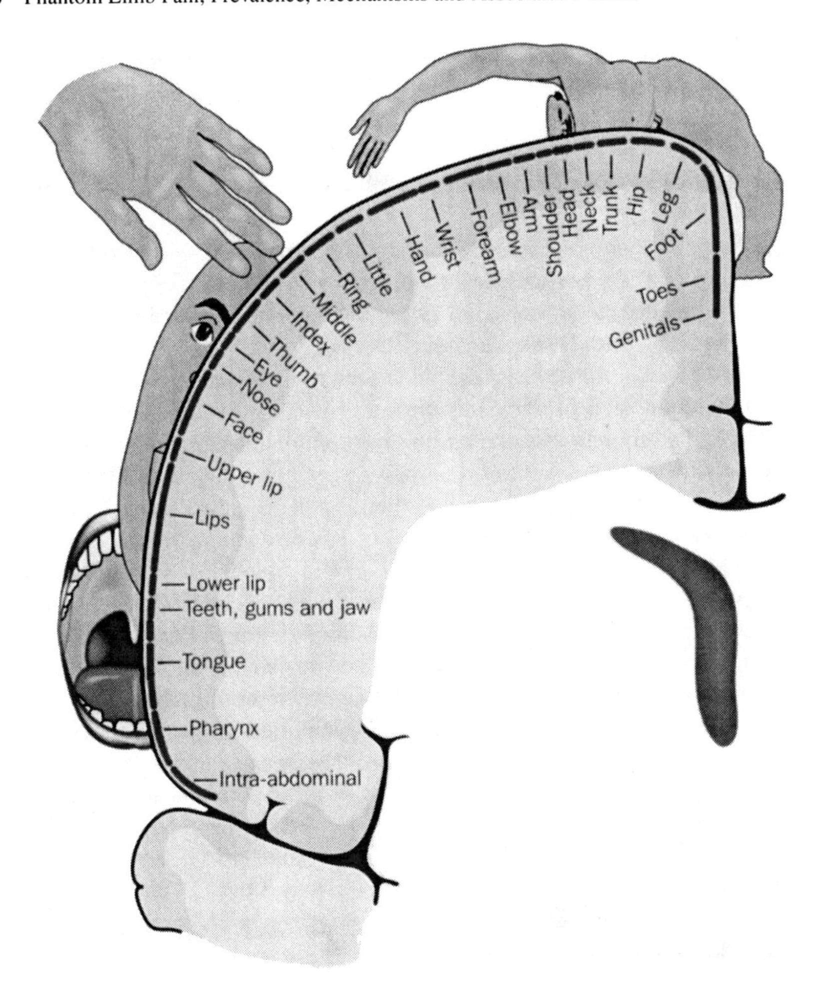

Fig. 10.2 Penfield map of the sensory homunculus

the cortical reorganisations are significantly reduced or return to the pre-amputation state (Chan et al. 2007; Knecht et al. 1998; Lotze et al. 1999; Weiss et al. 1999).

Other brain areas are also implicated in PLP development or maintenance: these are the motor cortex (Condes-Lara et al. 2000; Dettmers et al. 2001; Hugdahl et al. 2001; Karl et al. 2001; Roux et al. 2001; Willoch et al. 2000), the thalamus (Davis et al. 1998; Lenz et al. 1998) and the vestibular region (Le Chapelain et al. 2001).

In summary, many different brain areas are under investigation for involvement in PLP development and maintenance. Much of the work has been done with upper limb amputees, and it remains to be confirmed that similar reorganisations occur in lower limb amputees. Such complexity and the presence of phenomena such as super-added sensations and the continued reports from amputees that their PLP is similar to their pre-amputation pain means that the concept of a neuronal memory playing a role in PLP will not go away.

10.1.2.4 Pain/Neuronal Memory and PLP

The idea of pain memory has been discussed in relation to PLP throughout the centuries (Wade 2008); however, work with animals and human experimentation to establish the link expanded within the 1990s (Hodges and Bender 1994; Katz 1992; Katz and Melzack 1990; Ramachandran 1998).

The animal model for neuropathic pains such as PLP is autotomy. Autotomy is the self-mutilation seen in rats, following nerve injury. If the sciatic and/or the saphenous nerves are resected, the rat will be seen to nibble and then chew off the toes and foot. It is postulated that this behaviour is associated with parasthesias similar to phantom sensations and PLP. Although it is recognised to have limitations (Kauppila 1998), autotomy is the most widely accepted animal model for PLP.

In an elaborate experiment, (Katz et al. 1991) found that rats sensitised by previous injury showed altered autotomy to those who only had their nerve resected. Injury was induced by heat, electrical or mechanical stimulation. The previously injured rats showed earlier onset ($p<0.04$) and increased autotomy ($p<0.002$). It was postulated that the injury produced changes within the central nervous system, which were crystallised (synaptically) as memories. These gave a propensity for pain symptomology following future noxious events that employed similar nerve pathways. Similar assumptions were made when formalin was injected into rats paws prior to nerve resection (Abad et al. 1998). Those rats that were resected 30 min following the painful injection were found to exhibit faster onset of autotomy than those that were resected at 60 min, 1 day, 3 days, 7 days and 14 days after injection ($p<0.05$). This suggests that severe pain at or near the time of amputation increases the risk of developing PLP.

In humans, much of the evidence is anecdotal. Pain memory is assumed in the subset of amputees who develop delayed onset PLP, which is 10–33% of cases (Schott 2001), and in those with super-added pain. However, there is one case which lends weight to the theory (Halligan et al. 1993). This was a lady who required amputation after having treatment for carpel tunnel syndrome, which had manifested as numbness and pain in the thumb and index finger. One year following uncomplicated surgery to correct the carpel tunnel, the lady needed an amputation of the same arm for an unrelated condition. PLP subsequently developed, and it was described as being similar to the pain associated with the carpel tunnel. When the phantom was mapped on her face, it was found that her thumb and index finger were missing, suggesting that the previous experience had influenced the cortical reorganisation.

However, in a prospective study, it was found that the pre-amputation and post-amputation pain intensities and descriptors were different (Richardson et al. 2007). Using 2-way repeated measures ANOVA, it was found that the pre-amputation pain was different in the total number of descriptors chosen and in the pattern of descriptors chosen at the two time points confirming previous findings (Nikolajsen et al.

1997b). These prospective comparative studies start to call to question the pain memory theory for PLP; however, so many amputees state that their PLP is similar to the pain that they had prior to the amputation, or to pains that they had in the limb at some time in the past, it cannot yet be ignored (Katz and Melzack 1990). This observation plus evidence and reports from amputees suggest that phantom phenomena are a result of the complex interaction between multiple areas and processes throughout the nervous system, and the theory that best describes this is the neuromatrix theory (Melzack 1993).

10.1.2.5 The Neuromatrix Theory

Robert Melzack first proposed this theory in 1993, and it has yet to be verified; however, the underlying premise that the brain has a genetically determined neurosignature which can be modified by sensory input and experience remains enticing. Central to the theory are neural loops between all the areas of the brain known to be involved in pain processing including the cortex, limbic system, the insula and the thalamus. Inputs into the system of loops interact with the neurosignature to produce an output (in this case a phantom +/– PLP). The fact that it is output reliant is crucial to Melzack's argument for the neuromatrix theory to generate phantom phenomena and can explain why some amputees do not get pain. It can also explain, through the neurosignature, why paraplegics and congenitally limb deficient individuals get phantom symptoms including PLP.

In order to explain phantom phenomena, Melzack postulated 3 brain systems working in symmetry. (Melzack 1992; Melzack 1993; Melzack 1989). The classical and established system of pain pathways where sensory pathways pass through the thalamus to the somatosensory cortex is the first system. The second system includes the reticular formation of the brain stem and the limbic system. It is known that emotional components of pain are integrated through the limbic system. Melzack suggests that the third system comprises the areas that help to determine the attribute known as "self." Classical neurology favours the parietal lobe in this role.

Any sensory information from the periphery is analysed, shared among the three systems and converted into an integrated output. In order for the neuromatrix to function for phantom phenomena, it must modulate the input by stamping its signature onto it. The output therefore takes account of the sensory input, the recognition of the "normal" condition while also recognising everything as "self."

One of the overriding requirements of the neuromatrix theory is the need for the neuromatrix itself to be "hardwired." Hardwiring implies that the neural connections making up the neuromatrix are stable and unchanging and are probably genetically determined. The synaptic strength of the hardwired system, however, can be modified by experience. Neuronal pathways will be strengthened or will decay/die dependent upon use. Neural pathways will therefore become dominant or recessive dependent upon somatosensory input. As there is a myriad of possible somatosensory inputs, there are an infinite number of possible variations that can be imposed upon the neuromatrix because of the experience of living.

The neuromatrix theory therefore incorporates a genetic engram and an experience element. Both are important, but they must co-exist for the neuromatrix to function. These two elements mean that all variations and types of phantom phenomena could be explained through differences in any one or a combination of the three elements of the neuromatrix. The theory was originally proposed to explain phantom phenomena as a whole rather than each individual sensation, and because of this, it also explains how and why phantom phenomena are interrelated. The concept of pain memory and the presence of phantom phenomena in the congenitally limb deficient are explained, making it on the whole a reasonable theory. Over time, however, it needs to be tested and modified until it fully explains the phenomena. Following this refinement, it is possible that aspects of cortical reorganisation and pain/neuronal memory will be included. Having a theory of PLP mechanism opens the possibility for treatment strategies.

10.1.2.6 Treatment of PLP

As Kate MacIver will explain, in her chapter later in this book, treatment of PLP has been problematic. All forms of medication and surgical management and complementary therapies have been tried with little success for the majority of PLP sufferers. This means that focus has turned to the potential to prevent PLP from occurring in the first place (Bloomquist 2001).

10.1.2.6.1 Pre-Emptive Treatment for PLP

Pre-emption seems valid theoretically when the evidence supporting the links between PLP, cortical reorganisation, autotomy behaviour in pre-treated rats and pain memory are reviewed alongside the neuromatrix theory (Baron et al. 1998; Katz 1997; Thompson 1998; Ramachandran and Hirstein 1998). The neuromatrix theory presupposes that PLP is created by the output from the neuromatrix. This output will be related to the input; hence the potential that modifying input couldreduce the likelihood that PLP will result.

10.1.2.6.1.1 Evidence in Support of Pre-Emption

Evidence in favour of pre-emption in humans comes from the use of nerve blocks, and epidural infusions. The first used a nerve sheath block of the sciatic or post-tibial nerve sutured into place during lower limb amputation (Fisher and Meller 1991). Eleven consecutive patients were enrolled and compared to 20 retrospective patients. Follow up was maintained for 1 year. The treatment group was found to require less morphine, ($p<0.0001$) and none developed PLP, although two got occasional parasthesias.

The use of epidurals followed. In the first trial, treatment commenced 24 h before the surgery ($n=13$) and continued for 3 days after amputation (Jahangiri et al. 1994). The control group ($n = 11$) received traditional on demand opioids. Seven days after the surgery, 3 of the test group had PLP (23%), while 9 (82%) of the control group had developed PLP ($p < 0.01$). At 6 months and at 1 year, there was still a significant difference between the groups ($p < 0.002$). Phantom sensation was also significantly reduced in the test group up to 1year after amputation ($p < 0.05$). The lack of a placebo group and high morbidity makes these findings difficult to assess.

Commencement time of epidural infusions has also been compared (Schug et al. 1995). Group 1 ($n = 8$) had an epidural started 24 h prior to surgery, group 2 ($n = 7$) had the epidural commenced during the surgery and group 3 ($n = 8$) were given a general anaesthetic and traditional post-operative analgesics. At the 1 year follow-up, only one of group 1, three of group 2 and six of group 3 had PLP. Group 1 were significantly less likely to have PLP than group 3 ($p < 0.05$), although the small numbers in this study give these comparisons a very high risk of bias.

10.1.2.6.1.2 Evidence Against Pre-Emption

Evidence against pre-emption arises from studies using nerve blocks, epidural infusions and intrathecal administrations. In a non-randomised study of 19 test subjects and 40 controls, a sciatic or post-tibial catheter was used to infuse 0.5% bupivicaine (Elizaga et al. 1994). The catheter was inserted at the time of surgery and was maintained for between 3 and 7 days following the amputation. There was a large attrition rate with data from only 9 test subjects being available at the 6-month follow-up. When compared to the 12 controls who had complete data, there was no significant difference for PLP, phantom sensations, stump pain, opioid use or length of stay. This may have been influenced by the poor method of control in the study and the high dropout rate.

A similar prospective study ($n = 6$) on upper limb amputees, using a 0.25% bupivicaine also proved to be inconclusive (Enneking et al. 1997).

Perhaps the most convincing evidence so far to refute the effects of pre-emption on PLP was a prospective randomised trial of 60 patients. Groups received either epidural bupivicaine (0.25%; 4–7 ml/h) along with morphine (0.16–0.28 mg/h), or placebo epidural infusion of saline alongside oral or intramuscular morphine (Nikolajsen et al. 1997a). All infusions were commenced before surgery (15–20.3 h, median 18 h) and were continued for a median 166 h (89.3–308.3 h) post-operatively. Follow-up continued for 1 year, and at no point was there a significant difference between the test group ($n = 29$) and the placebo group ($n = 31$) for PLP. Arguments against this study revolve around the potential un-blinding of the placebo group and the short average time that the epidural was commenced prior to surgery. Some argue that the epidural needs to be in situ a minimum of 24 h prior to the amputation.

A further prospective study ($n = 21$) compared a group having intrathecal bupivicaine +/– opioid for existing PLP ($n = 16$) or preventing PLP (Dahm et al. 1998). The results showed that once the infusion was discontinued, each group developed significant levels of PLP. Of the preventative group, 56% went on to develop PLP. This is consistent with usual levels seen in amputees. Ninety percent of those treated for existing PLP found that it recurred.

In a randomized prospective study comparing preoperative and postoperative epidural infusion of bupivicaine and diamorphine with intraoperative perineural bupivicaine and systemic morphine, no difference in PLP was found between the groups at 3 days and at 1 year (Lambert et al. 2001). The epidural was sited 24 h prior to the amputation and was found to be effective at controlling stump pain in the early post-operative stage ($p=0.01$), but ineffective at preventing PLP. This study had a large drop out mainly due to patient death (12 out of 30 within 6 months of the surgery), so the final calculations were performed on small numbers.

10.1.2.6.1.3 Pre-Emption – A Summary

As with all areas of debate within the topic of PLP, the evidence on pre-emption is conflicting. There seems to be some evidence to support the fact that pre-amputation pain is associated with PLP but little to support the contention that controlling the pain prevents PLP from occurring. It is possible, however, that the evidence to date has not given the detail required to conclusively prove the worth of pre-emption.

The major issue is one of timing: when the cortical reorganisation occurs and when pre-emption has to be given to prevent this reorganisation from happening. Certainly, there is the suggestion that for some, cortical reorganisation had already occurred at the time of surgery (Elizaga et al. 1994; Katz 1997), and could already have happened pre-operatively, especially in those who had pain for long periods of time before the amputation (Grusser et al. 2001). Overall , pre-emption continues to be the focus of attention for the management of PLP, though.

Perhaps the issue, which most inhibits our knowledge in this field, is the fact that pre-emption has focused solely on pain. It is possible to postulate that other physical or psychological attributes may influence the cortical reorganisations associated with PLP, and as a result, targeting these will also have the potential to pre-empt PLP.

It has been suggested that the pre-amputation discussion should mention PLP and its management and in doing so, may go some way to alleviating the onset or disablement of PLP (Sherman 1989). Others have advocated that knowledge of the patient, including their normal coping strategies, personality and family support (Butler et al. 1992; Hill 1995; Rounseville 1992) is important both as a predictor for the onset of PLP and as a potential to intervene to prevent it (Dernham 1986; Tomeno et al. 1998). Full elucidation of these traits and their relationship to chronic pain conditions including PLP has yet to be explained. With this in mind, the study of pre-emption of PLP requires a full knowledge of factors that are known to be associated with PLP. These factors need to be identifiable and available for alteration prior to amputation if PLP is to be prevented.

10.1.2.7 Factors Associated with PLP

The first extensive review of factors thought to predispose an amputee to the development of PLP divided them into physical and socio-psychological (Mouratoglou 1986; *see* Table 10.1).

Table 10.1 Factors predisposing an amputee to the development of phantom limb pain

Physical*	Sociopsychological*
Over 35 years of age	Unemployment
Loss of sensorimotor function	Retirement caused by amputation
War injured	Recurrent depression
Prolonged illness	High neuroticism scale
Prolonged pain prior to amputation	Psychosomatic symptoms
Pathology to stump	High "lie scale" score
A threat to life or the other limb	Social isolation
Prolonged stump pain	Compulsive self-reliant and rigid personality
Delay in the supply of a prosthesis	Cultural/class influence
Minimal use of prosthesis	

*Modified from Mouratoglou (1986)

This list highlights one major difficulty when attempting to look at factors associated with any condition. That is the "chicken and egg" scenario. Most, if not the entire list, could have been caused by, rather than contributing to, PLP. It should also be noted, however, that once present, these factors may assist in the prolongation or continuation of PLP, but may not have been part of the original cause. Other papers have striven to identify associated factors more rigorously taking into account the possibilities of confounding variables.

10.1.2.7.1 Psychosociocultural Factors

One part of a questionnaire used to explore all aspects of PLP asked amputees to identify anything that induced their PLP (Sherman et al. 1984). The following were the results :

- 48% weather.
- 8% prosthetic problems.
- 6% mental stress.
- 4% fatigue.
- 2% gut and back problems.
- 26% no idea.

This suggests that up to 26% of cases of PLP are of unknown and potentially of endogenous origin.

Endogenous aspects of PLP, for example, links between the aetiology of the amputation and PLP, have been investigated. Stepwise logistic regression was used in a group of 536 amputees from a limb-fitting centre (Dijkstra et al. 2002). This group were on average 18.8 years from amputation, and included upper and lower limb amputees. Risk factors identified were lower limb ($p=0.001$), bilateral amputation ($p=0.001$), Peripheral vascular disease/diabetes ($p=0.001$), distal amputation ($p=0.04$), presence of phantom sensation ($p=0.001$) and presence of stump pain ($p=0.001$).

In a sample of 92 amputees (58 Caucasian and 34 African-American or Puerto Rican), the presence of infection or gangrene prior to the amputation significantly increased the risk of developing PLP ($p<0.001$). Also, the presence of a blood clot appeared to predispose PLP but did not reach statistical significance (Weiss and Lindell 1996). Memory was relied upon for these results, so the findings, especially for medical details, must be treated with caution. In this sample, Caucasians were more likely to have PLP than non-Caucasians. This variation, like those found between American and British veterans (Sherman and Sherman 1983; Wartan et al. 1997), supports the argument that cultural elements also play a role in PLP development.

Emotional states, including anxiety and depression have long been suspected to predispose, trigger and/or maintain PLP (Davis 1993; Esquenazi 1993; Harwood et al. 1992; Herbener 1988; Ribbers et al. 1989; Sherman 1994). Evidence to support this suspicion though is scarce as in a group of 50 British war veterans, war memories did not set off PLP and although unhappy memories did increase the number of words chosen from the McGill Pain Questionnaire, the increase was not statistically significant (Machin and Williams 1998).

Also, no link between anxiety, depression and emotional adjustment including the grieving process and PLP could be identified (Fisher and Hanspal 1998). In this sample of 93 amputees, only 10 scored in the clinically significant range for anxiety, and this was mainly due to the fear of falling over. There was no significant difference between amputees with and without PLP; however, comparisons of this kind might miss individual variations.

In a further study, a 39-year-old woman with PLP completed a diary for 9 months (Hill et al. 1996). She was asked to identify all pain events and other events that were associated with her amputation and pain. The first month was used as a baseline. PLP was triggered on five occasions during the 9-month study. Two of these triggers could be attributed to emotional cues. The first one followed a discussion, with a friend, of the events leading up to her amputation. The other followed a television programme that showed a person using Entonox for a leg injury. As the woman had needed painful daily dressing of an ulcer on her leg for a substantial time prior to the amputation, and the fact that she used Entonox during those dressings, gave this drama a real life and an emotional edge for her. These emotional triggers were internalisations of an external stimulus. It is difficult, therefore, to determine if the trigger was endogenous, exogenous or a mixture of both.

A further complication is the finding that when faced with psychological stress, amputees with PLP react physiologically differently from those who do not experience PLP (Angrilli and Koster 2000). When asked to relate the amputation event, those with PLP showed increased heart rate and systolic blood pressure in comparison with those who did not have PLP. Pain was also exacerbated by the experience.

Various other studies have also shown that PLP, phantom sensation and stump pain are correlated, but no causal link has yet been made between them (Nikolajsen and Jensen 2001).

Pre-emption studies suggest that pain prior to amputation is thought to be related to PLP development, and many other studies hint that the psychosocial aspects of pre-amputation pain may be as important as its physical presence. What is clear is the different or altered biopsychosocial profiles between amputees with and without PLP could have occurred following the amputation or pre-existed before the amputation. It is important, therefore, to monitor biopsychosocial parameters prior to and following amputation, which could only be possible in elective cases and has only been attempted once.

A group of 59 people who had been scheduled for major lower limb amputation because of peripheral vascular disease were chosen for the study (Richardson et al. 2007). Once the decision to amputate was made, each participant was interviewed and followed up 6-months post-amputation. The pre-amputation and post-amputation conditions of those who had PLP were compared with those of the amputees who did not develop PLP.

The vast majority of survivors at 6-months had PLP (78%); hence the statistical comparisons had to be performed on unequal groups; however, some interesting discoveries were made. Although some weak links were found between pre-amputation pain and the presence of PLP, by far, the strongest link was pre-amputation coping style. Those participants who were passive copers prior to the amputation had a significantly higher risk of developing PLP than those who were active copers ($p=0.00$; OR 4.6; CI 3.5–25.0). The major contributor to the passive coping style was high levels of pre-amputation catastrophizing, which was also found to vary between those with and without PLP ($p=0.02$; OR 3.3; CI 1.7–14.9). Findings from other studies have suggested that catastrophizing is a key factor in developing and maintaining other chronic pain conditions. By implication, the neuronal components utilised in the process of coping may well be associated with those used within pain pathways. This means that the neuromatrix could be influenced by the coping style with the output being PLP.

Future studies on pre-emption, therefore, need to focus on psychological factors specifically coping style alongside pain reduction before it can be effective.

In summary, PLP occurs in adults, children and congenitally limbless individuals. The incidence is between 50% and 78% in adults, and as treatment so far has been unsuccessful, focus has shifted to the potential to prevent it from occurring in the first place. Such pre-emption needs targets, and there is still work to do to understand how PLP develops and to identify internal factors within an individual that predispose them to and maintains PLP. Interest has therefore focused upon finding ways to reverse peri-amputation cortical reorganisations and modifying coping style.

References

Abad F, Feria M, Sanchez A, Gonzalez Mora JL (1998) Autotomy in rats following peripheral nerve transection is attenuated by preceding formalin injections into the same limb. Neurosci Lett 243(1–3):125–128

Angrilli A, Koster U (2000) Psychophysiological stress responses in amputees with and without phantom limb pain. Physiol Behav 68(5):699–706

Baron R, Wasner G, Lindner V (1998) Optimal treatment of phantom limb pain in the elderly. Drugs Aging 12(5):361–376

Battrum DE, Gutmann JL (1996) Phantom tooth pain: a diagnosis of exclusion. Int Endod J 29(3):190–194

Biley FC (2001) Phantom bladder sensations: A new concern for stoma care workers. Br J Nurs 10(19):1290–1296

Bloomquist T (2001) Amputation and phantom limb pain: a pain-prevention model. AANA J 69(3):211–217

Butler DJ, Turkal NW, Seidl JJ (1992) Amputation: preoperative psychological preparation. J Am Board Fam Pract 5(1):69–73

Chan BL, Witt R, Charrow AP, Magee A, Howard R, Pasquina P (2007) Mirror therapy for phantom limb pain. N Engl J Med 357(21):2206–2207

Coderre TJ, Katz J (1997) Peripheral and central hyperexcitability: Differential signs and symptoms in persistent pain. Behav Brain Sci 20(3):404–412

Condes-Lara M, Barrios FA, Romo JR, Rojas R, Salgado P, Sanchez-Cortazar J (2000) Brain somatic representation of phantom and intact limb: A fMRI study case report. Eur J Pain 4(3):239–245

Dahm PO, Nitrescu PV, Appelgren LK, Curelanu ID (1998) Long-term intrathecal infusiion of opioid and/or bupivicaine in the prophylaxis and treatment of phantom limb pain. Neuromodulation 1(3):111–128

Davis RW (1993) Phantom sensation, phantom pain, and stump pain. Arch Phys Med Rehabil 74(1):79–91

Davis KD, Kiss ZH, Luo L, Tasker RR, Lozano AM, Dostrovsky JO (1998) Phantom sensations generated by thalamic microstimulation. Nature 391(6665):385–387

Dernham P (1986) Phantom limb pain. Geriatr Nurs 7(1):34–37

Dettmers C, Adler T, Rzanny R, van Schayck R, Gaser C, Weiss T, Miltner WH, Bruckner L, Weiller C (2001) Increased excitability in the primary motor cortex and supplementary motor area in patients with phantom limb pain after upper limb amputation. Neurosci Lett 307(2):109–112

Dijkstra PU, Geertzen JH, Stewart R, van der Schans CP (2002) Phantom pain and risk factors: a multivariate analysis. J Pain Symptom Manage 24(6):578–585

Dijkstra PU, Rietman JS, Geertzen JHB (2007) Phantom breast sensations and phantom breast pain: A 2-year prospective study and a methodological analysis of literature. Eur J Pain 11(1):99–108

DOH (2008) UK department of health, hospital episode statistics, vol 2008, London

Ehde DM, Czerniecki JM, Smith DG, Campbell KM, Edwards WT, Jensen MP, Robinson LR (2000) Chronic phantom sensations, phantom pain, residual limb pain, and other regional pain after lower limb amputation. Arch Phys Med Rehabil 81(8):1039–1044

Elizaga AM, Smith DG, Sharar SR, Edwards WT, Hansen ST Jr (1994) Continuous regional analgesia by intraneural block: Effect on postoperative opioid requirements and phantom limb pain following amputation. J Rehabil Res Dev 31(3):179–187

Enneking FK, Scarborough MT, Radson EA (1997) Local anesthetic infusion through nerve sheath catheters for analgesia following upper extremity amputation. Clinical report. Reg Anesth 22(4):351–356

Esquenazi A (1993) Geriatric amputee rehabilitation. Clin Geriatr Med 9(4):731–743

Fainsinger RL, de Gara C, Perez GA (2000) Amputation and the prevention of phantom pain. J Pain Symptom Manage 20(4):308–312

Finnoff J (2001) Differentiation and treatment of phantom sensation, phantom pain, and residual-limb pain. J Am Podiatr Med Assoc 91(1):23–33

Fisher CM (1999) Phantom erection after amputation of penis. Case description and review of the relevant literature on phantoms. Can J Neurol Sci 26(1):53–56

Fisher K, Hanspal RS (1998) Phantom pain, anxiety, depression, and their relation in consecutive patients with amputated limbs: case reports. BMJ 316(7135):903–904

Fisher A, Meller Y (1991) Continuous postoperative regional analgesia by nerve sheath block for amputation surgery – a pilot study. Anesth Analg 72(3):300–303

Flor H, Elbert T, Knecht S, Wienbruch C, Pantev C, Birbaumer N, Larbig W, Taub E (1995) Phantom-limb pain as a perceptual correlate of cortical reorganization following arm amputation. Nature 375(6531):482–484

Grusser SM, Winter C, Schaefer M, Fritzsche K, Benhidjeb T, Tunn P, Schlag PM and Flor H (2001) Perceptual phenomena after unilateral arm amputation: a pre-post surgical comparison. Neuroscience letters. 302(1):13–16

Halligan PW, Marshall JC, Wade DT, Davey J, Morrison D (1993) Thumb in cheek? Sensory reorganization and perceptual plasticity after limb amputation. Neuroreport 4(3):233–236

Hanowell ST, Kennedy SF (1979) Phantom tongue pain and causalgia: Case presentation and treatment. Anesth Analg 58(5):436–438

Harwood DD, Hanumanthu S, Stoudemire A (1992) Pathophysiology and management of phantom limb pain. Gen Hosp Psychiatry 14(2):107–118

Herbener D (1988) The phantom limb phenomenon. Physician Assist 12(7):57–58

Hill EM (1995) Perioperative management of patients with vascular disease. AACN Clin Issues 6(4):547–561

Hill A (1999) Phantom limb pain: a review of the literature on attributes and potential mechanisms. J Pain Symptom Manage 17(2):125–142

Hill A, Niven CA, Knussen C (1996) Pain memories in phantom limbs: a case study. Pain 66(2–3):381–384

Hodges C, Bender L (1994) Phantom pain: A critical review of the proposed mechanisms. Br J Occup Ther 57(6):209–212 35 ref

Houghton AD, Nicholls G, Houghton AL, Saadah E, McColl L (1994) Phantom pain: natural history and association with rehabilitation. Ann R Coll Surg Engl 76(1):22–25

Hugdahl K, Rosen G, Ersland L, Lundervold A, Smievoll AI, Barndon R, Thomsen T (2001) Common pathways in mental imagery and pain perception: an fMRI study of a subject with an amputated arm. Scand J Psychol 42(3):269–275

Hunter JP, Katz J, Davis KD (2003) The effect of tactile and visual sensory inputs on phantom limb awareness. Brain 126(Pt 3):579–589

Jahangiri M, Jayatunga AP, Bradley JW, Dark CH (1994) Prevention of phantom pain after major lower limb amputation by epidural infusion of diamorphine, clonidine and bupivacaine [see comment]. Ann R Coll Surg Engl 76(5):324–326

Jensen TS, Nikolajsen L (1999) Phantom pain and other phenomena after amputation. In Wall, P. and Melzack, R. (Eds) The textbook of pain. Churchill Livingstone. London.

Jensen TS, Nikolajsen L (2000) Pre-emptive analgesia in post-amputation pain: an update. Prog Pain Res 129:493–503

Jensen TS, Krebs B, Nielsen J, Rasmussen P (1983) Phantom limb, phantom pain and stump pain in amputees during the first 6 months following limb amputation. Pain 17(3):243–256

Jensen TS, Krebs B, Nielsen J, Rasmussen P (1985) Immediate and long-term phantom limb pain in amputees: Incidence, clinical characteristics and relationship to pre-amputation limb pain. Pain 21(3):267–278

Kalauokalani D, Loeser JD (1999) Phantom limb pain. IASP Press, Seattle

Karl A, Birbaumer N, Lutzenberger W, Cohen LG, Flor H (2001) Reorganization of motor and somatosensory cortex in upper extremity amputees with phantom limb pain. J Neurosci 21(10):3609–3618

Katz J (1992) Psychophysical correlates of phantom limb experience. J Neurol Neurosurg Psychiatry 55(9):811–821

Katz J (1997) Phantom limb pain. Lancet 350(9088):1338–1339

Katz J, Melzack R (1990) Pain "memories" in phantom limbs: review and clinical observations. Pain 43(3):319–336

Katz J, Vaccarino AL, Coderre TJ, Melzack R (1991) Injury prior to neurectomy alters the pattern of autotomy in rats. Behavioral evidence of central neural plasticity [see comment]. Anesthesiology 75(5):876–883

Kauppila T (1998) Correlation between autotomy-behavior and current theories of neuropathic pain. Neurosci Biobehav Rev 23(1):111–129

Knecht S, Henningsen H, Elbert T, Flor H, Hohling C, Pantev C, Taub E (1996) Reorganizational and perceptional changes after amputation. Brain 119(Pt 4):1213–1219

Knecht S, Henningsen H, Hohling C, Elbert T, Flor H, Pantev C, Taub E (1998) Plasticity of plasticity? Changes in the pattern of perceptual correlates of reorganization after amputation. Brain 121(Pt 4):717–724

Knox DJ, McLeod BJ, Goucke CR (1995) Acute phantom limb pain controlled by ketamine. Anaesth Intensive Care 23(5):620–622

Kooijman CM, Dijkstra PU, Geertzen JH, Elzinga A, van der Schans CP (2000) Phantom pain and phantom sensations in upper limb amputees: An epidemiological study. Pain 87(1):33–41

Krane EJ, Heller LB (1995) The prevalence of phantom sensation and pain in pediatric amputees. J Pain Symptom Manage 10(1):21–29

Lambert A, Dashfield A, Cosgrove C, Wilkins D, Walker A, Ashley S (2001) Randomized prospective study comparing preoperative epidural and intraoperative perineural analgesia for the prevention of postoperative stump and phantom limb pain following major amputation. Reg Anesth Pain Med 26(4):316–321

Le Chapelain L, Beis JM, Paysant J, Andre JM (2001) Vestibular caloric stimulation evokes phantom limb illusions in patients with paraplegia. Spinal Cord 39(2):85–87

Lenz FA, Garonzik IM, Zirh TA, Dougherty PM (1998) Neuronal activity in the region of the thalamic principal sensory nucleus (ventralis caudalis) in patients with pain following amputations. Neuroscience 86(4):1065–1081

Lotze M, Grodd W, Birbaumer N, Erb M, Huse E, Flor H (1999) Does use of a myoelectric prosthesis prevent cortical reorganization and phantom limb pain? Nat Neurosci 2(6):501–502

Lyth H (1995) Orthopaedics: Invisible problem. Nurs Times 91(19):38–40

Machin P, Williams AC de C (1998) Stiff upper lip: coping strategies of World War II veterans with phantom limb pain. Clin J Pain 14(4):290–294

McCartney CJL, Charles DHM, Cooper GG, Chambers WA, Smith WCS (1999) Pain and disability following lower limb amputation – a quantitative and qualitative study. Pain Clin 11(4):293–300

McMahon G (1998) Phantom limb pain following amputation. Paediatr Nurs 10(6):22–25

Melzack R (1989) Labat lecture. Phantom limbs. Reg Anesth 14(5):208–211

Melzack R (1992) Phantom limbs. Sci Am 266(4):120–126

Melzack R (1993) Pain: past, present and future. Can J Exp Psychol 47(4):615–629

Melzack R, Loeser JD (1978) Phantom body pain in paraplegics: evidence for a central "pattern generating mechanism" for pain. Pain 4(3):195–210

Melzack R, Israel R, Lacroix R, Schultz G (1997) Phantom limbs in people with congenital limb deficiency or amputation in early childhood. Brain 120(Pt 9):1603–1620

Montoya P, Larbig W, Grulke N, Flor H, Taub E, Birbaumer N (1997) The relationship of phantom limb pain to other phantom limb phenomena in upper extremity amputees. Pain 72(1–2):87–93

Mouratoglou VM (1986) Amputees and phantom limb pain: a literature review. Physiother Pract 2(4):177–185

Nikolajsen L, Jensen T (2000) Phantom limb pain. Curr Rev Pain 4(2):166–170

Nikolajsen L, Jensen TS (2001) Phantom limb pain. Br J Anaesth 87(1):107–116

Nikolajsen L, Ilkjaer S, Christensen JH, Kroner K, Jensen TS (1997a) Randomised trial of epidural bupivacaine and morphine in prevention of stump and phantom pain in lower-limb amputation [see comment]. Lancet 350(9088):1353–1357

Nikolajsen L, Ilkjaer S, Kroner K, Christensen JH, Jensen TS (1997b) The influence of preamputation pain on postamputation stump and phantom pain. Pain 72(3):393–405

Patterson JW (1994) Banishing phantom pain. Nursing 24(9):64

Pohjolainen T (1991) A clinical evaluation of stumps in lower limb amputees. Prosthet Orthot Int 15(3):178–184

Ramachandran VS (1998) Consciousness and body image: Lessons from phantom limbs, Capgras syndrome and pain asymbolia. Philos Trans R Soc Lond B Biol Sci 353(1377):1851–1859
Ramachandran VS, Hirstein W (1998) The perception of phantom limbs. The D.O. Hebb lecture. Brain 121:1603–1630
Ramachandran VS, Rogers-Ramachandran D (1996) Synaesthesia in phantom limbs induced with mirrors. Proc Biol Sci 263(1369):377–386
Ramachandran VS, Stewart M, Rogers-Ramachandran DC (1992) Perceptual correlates of massive cortical reorganization. Neuroreport 3(7):583–586
Ribbers G, Mulder T, Rijken R (1989) The phantom phenomenon: a critical review. Int J Rehabil Res 12(2):175–186
Richardson C, Glenn S, Nurmikko T, Horgan M (2006) Incidence of phantom phenomena including phantom limb pain 6 months after major lower limb amputation in patients with peripheral vascular disease. Clin J Pain 22(4):353–358
Richardson C, Glenn S, Horgan M, Nurmikko T (2007) A prospective study of factors associated with the presence of phantom limb pain six months after major lower limb amputation in patients with peripheral vascular disease. J Pain 8(10):793–801
Rounseville C (1992) Phantom limb pain: the ghost that haunts the amputee. Orthop Nurs 11(2):67–71
Roux FE, Ibarrola D, Lazorthes Y, Berry I (2001) Virtual movements activate primary sensorimotor areas in amputees: report of three cases. Neurosurgery 49(3):736–741 discussion 741–742
Schott GD (2001) Delayed onset and resolution of pain: some observations and implications. Brain 124(Pt 6):1067–1076
Schug SA, Burrell R, Payne J, Tester P (1995) Pre-emptive epidural analgesia may prevent phantom limb pain [comment]. Reg Anesth 20(3):256
Sherman RA (1989) Stump and phantom limb pain. Neurol Clin 7(2):249–264
Sherman RA (1994) Phantom limb pain. Mechanism-based management. Clin Podiatr Med Surg 11(1):85–106
Sherman RA, Sherman CJ (1983) Prevalence and characteristics of chronic phantom limb pain among American veterans. Results of a trial survey. Am J Phys Med 62(5):227–238
Sherman RA, Sherman CJ, Parker L (1984) Chronic phantom and stump pain among American veterans: results of a survey. Pain 18(1):83–95
Sherman RA, Griffin VD, Evans CB, Grana AS (1992) Temporal relationships between changes in phantom limb pain intensity and changes in surface electromyogram of the residual limb. Int J Psychophysiol 13(1):71–77
Smith DG, Ehde DM, Legro MW, Reiber GE, del Aguila M, Boone DA (1999) Phantom limb, residual limb, and back pain after lower extremity amputations. Clin Orthop Relat Res 361:29–38
Stannard CF (1993) Phantom limb pain [see comment]. Br J Hosp Med 50(10):583–584
Thompson HM (1998) Pain after amputation: is prevention better than cure? Br J Anaesth 80(4):415–416
Tomeno B, Anract P, Ouaknine M (1998) Psychological management, prevention and treatment of phantom pain after amputations for tumours. Int Orthop 22(3):205–208
Wade NJ (2008) Beyond body experiences: Phantom limbs, pain and the locus of sensation. Cortex, 45(2):243–255
Wartan SW, Hamann W, Wedley JR, McColl I (1997) Phantom pain and sensation among British veteran amputees. Br J Anaesth 78(6):652–659
Weinstein SM (1998) Phantom limb pain and related disorders. Neurol Clin 16(4):919–936
Weinstein SM, Anderson MD (1994) Phantom pain. Oncology 8(3):65–70 discussion 70, 73–74
Weir Mitchell S (1871) Phantom limbs. Mag Pop Lit Sci 8:563–569
Weiss SA, Lindell B (1996) Phantom limb pain and etiology of amputation in unilateral lower extremity amputees. J Pain Symptom Manage 11(1):3–17
Weiss T, Miltner WH, Adler T, Bruckner L, Taub E (1999) Decrease in phantom limb pain associated with prosthesis-induced increased use of an amputation stump in humans. Neurosci Lett 272(2):131–134

Wesolowski JA, Lema MJ (1993) Phantom limb pain. Reg Anesth 18(2):121–127
Wilkins KL, McGrath PJ, Finley GA, Katz J (1998) Phantom limb sensations and phantom limb pain in child and adolescent amputees. Pain 78(1):7–12
Wilkins KL, McGrath PJ, Finley GA, Katz J (2004) Prospective diary study of nonpainful and painful phantom sensations in a preselected sample of child and adolescent amputees reporting phantom limbs. Clin J Pain 20(5):293–301
Williams AM, Deaton SB (1997) Phantom limb pain: elusive, yet real. Rehabil Nurs 22(2):73–77
Williamson VC (1992) Amputation of the lower extremity: an overview. Orthop Nurs 11(2):55–65
Willoch F, Rosen G, Tolle TR, Oye I, Wester HJ, Berner N, Schwaiger M, Bartenstein P (2000) Phantom limb pain in the human brain: unraveling neural circuitries of phantom limb sensations using positron emission tomography. Ann Neurol 48(6):842–849
Yetser EA (1996) Helping the patient through the experience of an amputation. Orthop Nurs 15(6):45–49

Chapter 11
Management of Phantom Limb Pain

Kate MacIver and Donna Lloyd

Abstract This chapter provides a comprehensive overview of the management of chronic phantom limb pain (PLP) as it relates to the patient in the prosthesis clinic. The chapter begins with phantom pain assessment. Pharmacological therapies commonly used in the treatment of PLP will be discussed, with a review of the literature relating to success or otherwise of these medications. The side-effects of the drugs are highlighted, and the necessary advice to be given to patients is provided. What follows is a review of non-pharmacological therapies, beginning with Neuromodulation (TENS, spinal cord and deep brain stimulation). Psychological aspects of treatment are identified – how to recognise psychological distress; how to know when to refer on for psychological treatment and useful psychological interventions. The chapter concludes with suggestions for the holistic management of patients suffering from PLP. The role of mental imagery is highlighted.

11.1 Introduction

Despite the fact that phantom limb pain (PLP) has been recognised as a distinct pain syndrome for over a hundred years, it still remains a challenging problem for the clinician and the patient alike. Standard drug therapies have limited benefit, and there are no comprehensive randomised clinical trials to guide best practice (Nikolajsen and Jensen 2006). In common with other chronic pain syndromes, the causes and maintenance of PLP may be due to a complex array of factors, mediated by the peripheral and central nervous systems and further complicated by psychological factors (Flor 2002). Given the dearth of clinical trials to assess the effect of analgesic management of PLP, and since PLP is accepted to be a neuropathic pain (i.e., pain originating in the peripheral or central nervous system) it is useful to examine the literature relating to the management of neuropathic pain in general, in order to come to a consensus on how to help the patient (Nikolajsen and Jensen 2006).

K. MacIver (✉)
Pain Research Institute in Liverpool, Liverpool, UK
e-mail: k.maciver@liverpool.ac.uk

C. Murray (ed.), *Amputation, Prosthesis Use, and Phantom Limb Pain: An Interdisciplinary Perspective*, DOI 10.1007/978-0-387-87462-3_11,

In the previous chapter the complexity of the mechanisms of the generation and maintenance of PLP was highlighted. Perhaps it is this complexity which makes PLP so difficult to treat, with contributions from long-standing pain pre-amputation, the generation of a cortical "memory" for pain, increased excitability of nerve fibres at the peripheral and central level, reorganisation of the cortical representation of the missing body part and psychosocial issues (Flor 2002).

Therapeutic attempts to treat phantom pain range from simple analgesics, strong opiates, antidepressants and anticonvulsants to surgical techniques such as refashioning of the stump, and neurosurgery including spinal cord stimulation (SCS) and deep brain stimulation (Halbert et al. 2002). There is now considerable interest in the use of novel therapies such as imagined movement of the missing limb (MacIver et al. 2008) or laterality recognition and graded motor imagery (Moseley 2006) as a means of relieving PLP.

11.2 Pain Assessment

PLP is common in amputees and notoriously difficult to treat. People with amputation may begin to suffer from phantom pain immediately after surgery, or not until many years have passed. However, it seems that health professionals may not ask patients about the existence of PLP, nor offer treatment – for example, a study by Sherman et al. (1984) found that 78% of people questioned complained of pain in the missing limb but only 19% of pain sufferers had been offered treatment, and of these, only 1.1% had benefited. Many sufferers never ask for treatment. A more recent study by Kooijman et al. (2000) of upper limb amputees found a similar problem – only a minority of respondents had been treated for PLP, despite an incidence in this study of 51%.

Inadequate treatment of any persistent pain affects quality of life by decreasing work opportunities and increasing functional impairment and psychological distress (McCarberg and Stanos 2008). This is particularly applicable in the case of phantom pain, where the patient already has to deal with the impairment of amputation, and where PLP and stump pain may interfere with prosthesis use and rehabilitation.

Therefore, the first step to successful management of PLP is to ascertain the nature and extent of the problem in each individual, and the first requirement in this is to ensure that the patient knows that health professionals and caregivers accept their pain as real. PLP may be present immediately after amputation, or may develop after several years, so patients should be asked at each contact if pain is an issue.

Having acknowledged the presence of PLP, the next step is to establish the nature of the pain and how much it interferes with everyday life. McCarberg and Stanos (2008), in a useful review of current pain assessment strategies, comment on the "PQRST" acronym, proposed by the American Pain Society, to help clinicians remember the important factors in comprehensive pain assessment.

- *P* Provocative – i.e., what factors trigger the pain? In PLP, for example, this may be applying or removing the prosthesis, scratching the head (in the case of arm amputation) or passing urine (in the case of leg amputation).

- *Q* Quality of pain – what descriptors does the patient use to describe PLP? PLP is commonly described as shooting, burning, squeezing (Nikolajsen and Jensen 2001). The McGill Pain Questionnaire, either the standard or short form, is a reliable, validated tool to evaluate subjective pain experience, giving the patient the choice of words to describe their pain (Melzack and Katz 2006).
- *R* Region of pain – many amputees suffer from PLP, stump pain and other pains, such as low back pain (common after leg amputation) and it is helpful to distinguish one from the other prior to beginning treatment.
- *S* Severity of pain. The study by Kooijman et al. (2000) found an incidence of PLP in 51% of their cohort. Of these, 64% had pain which was moderate to severe and 36% mild to moderate. The degree of perceived suffering will influence the need for intervention.
- *T* Temporal. The onset of PLP, how often it occurs (it varies amongst patients from continuous to rarely; Flor 2002); whether it is more or less severe as time goes on. Re-assessment of pain at each clinic visit is essential, not only to investigate the natural pain history of each individual, but also to assess the efficacy of treatment.

Patients can keep a pain diary, using simple Numerical Rating Scores (NRS 0–10 where 0=no pain and 10=the worst pain imaginable) or a Visual Analogue Scale (VAS) which is a 10 cm line measuring from 0 (no pain) at one end to 10 (worst imaginable pain) at the other end. For young children or those with cognitive difficulties, a simple Faces Pain Rating Scale allows the respondent to point to the facial expression which best describes their current pain experience (McCarberg and Stanos 2008). Consistency is of course important, with the same assessment tool being used throughout treatment.

11.3 Pharmacological Management of PLP

Most pharmacological treatments for PLP are ineffective and are not pain mechanism-based (Flor 2002). It is impossible to give clear treatment guidelines based on good evidence, as that good evidence does not exist (Nikolajsen and Jensen 2001). There is a dearth of randomised, controlled trials evaluating the efficacy of analgesia and surgical interventions (Flor 2002). Therefore, the following paragraphs on pharmacological treatments will, where necessary, evaluate those treatments from the literature relating to neuropathic pain.

11.4 The World Health Organisation Analgesic Ladder

The WHO analgesic ladder was developed to provide a logical stepwise approach to cancer pain (WHO 1996), beginning with simple analgesics such as paracetamol and moving up to more potent analgesia such as morphine, as the need arose (Mishra et al. 2008). The original 3-step ladder consists of the prescription of non-opiate analgesia (paracetamol, non-steroidal analgesics) for mild-moderate pain; weak opiates for mild-moderate pain and strong opiates for moderate-severe pain

(Grond et al. 1999). It has been adapted to a 4-step ladder to incorporate the use of adjuvant medications (for example anti-depressants or anti-convulsants) and interventions (such as nerve blocks) which may be necessary for the management of the neuropathic element of cancer pain (Grond et al. 1999). Mishra et al. (2008) used this 4-step ladder in a small study of phantom pain related to limb amputation for cancer. They found no reduction in phantom pain when step 1 (non-opiate medication) was in use, and although the best results were obtained with the use of morphine (Step 3, strong opiate) there was no significant difference between Step 2 and Step 3. All these patients were also prescribed adjuvant medication – 60% on amitriptyline and 40% on gabapentin, but the effects of these drugs were not evaluated. Despite the limitations of this study (small numbers, non-experimental, no control group) it can be seen that there was no benefit from the WHO Step 1 (non-opiates paracetamol and ibuprofen), that opiates themselves may have a beneficial effect on PLP, and confirms the traditional view that neuropathic pain is not helped by standard non-opiate analgesics (Backonja 2002).

11.5 Antidepressant Therapy

Evidence-based recommendations for the management of neuropathic pain suggest certain antidepressants as a first-line treatment (Dworkin et al. 2007). These include the tricyclic antidepressants such as amitriptyline or nortriptyline, selective serotonin reuptake inhibitors (SSRIs), such as fluoxetine and the selective serotonin and noradrenaline reuptake inhibitors (SSNRIs), such as venlafaxine or duloxetine. The Cochrane library review of the use of antidepressants for neuropathic pain (Saarto and Wiffen 2007) does not include a comprehensive randomised controlled trial of antidepressant therapy for PLP, but a summary of 61 trials of 20 antidepressants concluded that tricyclic antidepressants may have a moderately beneficial effect in 1 out of 3 patients, with the best evidence available for the use of amitriptyline. A small ($N=39$) placebo-controlled study of the use of amitriptyline for relief of PLP had a negative result (Robinson et al. 2004). There is limited evidence for the beneficial effects of SSRIs, and the newer SSNRIs have not been clinically proven for the management of central pain.

We may be able to conclude, therefore, that tricyclic antidepressants may be helpful as a first line pharmacological therapy for the management of PLP, although larger Randomised Controlled Trials (RCT) are needed.

11.5.1 Side-Effects

11.5.1.1 Tricyclics

Heart arrhythmias and heart block occasionally occur with treatment with tricyclics (particularly amitriptyline), and should not be prescribed to people with known heart disease. Patients over 40 years of age should have a preliminary electrocardiogram

(Dworkin et al. 2007). Other common side-effects include dry mouth, sedation, blurred vision, urinary retention and sweating (BNF 2008).

11.5.1.2 SSRIs

Common side-effects include nausea, vomiting, diarrhoea, constipation, anorexia, rash (which may be serious and require immediate withdrawal of the drug), dry mouth and sedation (BNF 2008).

11.5.1.3 SSNRIs

The side-effect profile is similar to that of the other antidepressants. These drugs should be avoided in patients with heart disease, hypertension and glaucoma. Common side-effects include constipation, nausea, hypertension, palpitations, insomnia and nervousness.

11.5.2 Advice to Patients

Patients should understand that these drugs are being prescribed for pain management rather than depression (and indeed they are normally used at a lower dose than that required for depression treatment; Saarto and Wiffen 2007). It may take several days for the full effect to be realised. Patients should be started on a low dose, which may be titrated to the required dose (which is dependent on the individual drug) over several days or weeks to minimise side-effects. Patients will need to make a decision regarding continuing treatment based on a balance between benefit and unwanted effects. If the drug is to be discontinued, the dose should be slowly tapered over a few weeks, to reduce the risk of withdrawal symptoms such as sweating, anxiety or headache (BNF 2008). Patients who suffer from untoward drowsiness should avoid driving or using heavy machinery. Alcohol should be used with caution.

11.6 Anticonvulsant Therapy

Anticonvulsants, developed primarily for the prevention and treatment of convulsions in epilepsy, have been used for many years to treat neuropathic pain (Bone et al. 2002). The older anticonvulsant carbamazepine is most commonly used for the treatment of trigeminal neuralgia (Wiffen et al. 2005) and there are no clinical trials evaluating its efficacy in PLP. The common side-effect of cognitive impairment limits the value of this drug (BNF 2008).

The first-line anticonvulsant therapy for the management of neuropathic pain is gabapentin and its closely related counterpart pregabalin (Dworkin et al. 2007), and both these drugs are commonly given to patients with PLP. A small RCT by

Bone et al. (2002) demonstrated the superior analgesic qualities of gabapentin over placebo with 6 weeks of therapy. In common with the antidepressants, dose titration of both these drugs should be slow, as should withdrawal.

11.6.1 Side-Effects

Gabapentin has been in use for several years, and is generally well tolerated (Dworkin et al. 2007). Common side-effects include sedation, dry mouth, diarrhoea or constipation, changes in appetite, peripheral oedema and ataxia.

Pregabalin is a newer drug, so its long-term safety profile is not yet known (Dworkin et al. 2007). The side-effect profile is similar to that of gabapentin.

11.6.2 Advice to Patients

Patients should understand that they are being given these drugs for pain management and not epilepsy. They may need to wait several days or weeks, until the correct dose is reached, before they notice any benefit. Side-effects may be prominent at first and then reduce over time. Patients who suffer from untoward drowsiness should avoid driving or using heavy machinery. Alcohol should be used with caution.

11.7 Other Drugs

Opiate analgesics, including tramadol, have been shown to be efficacious in treating neuropathic pain. A double-blind, placebo-controlled crossover trial comparing morphine to mexilitine showed morphine to be more effective for the management of post-amputation pain, although this group did not differentiate stump pain from PLP in their study design. A case series of 12 patients with defined PLP showed a significant positive response to morphine (Huse et al. 2001). The long-term use of morphine may be limited by its side-effect profile (constipation, nausea, cognitive deficit, itching) and its negative status.

Memantine and ketamine have also been found to be ineffective in the management and prevention of chronic PLP (Maier et al. 2003; Schley et al. 2008).

11.8 Conclusion of Pharmacological Therapies

There is no outstanding effective drug for the treatment of PLP. This is complicated by the fact that there are no large clinical trials related to PLP. However, antidepressants such as amitriptyline, and anticonvulsants such as gabapentin and pregabalin have a proven effect for the management of other neuropathic pain syndromes, and might be tried in PLP sufferers, either alone or in combination (Dworkin et al. 2007), even if not specifically licensed for this purpose. Morphine has been shown to have some effect in the management of PLP, but trials are small. Dose-dependent side-effects in all these drugs may limit efficacy.

Dworkin et al. (2007) recommend that gabapentin or amitriptyline should be the first-line treatment in neuropathic pain – if the first one does not work, then switch to the other one.

11.9 Non-Pharmacological Therapy for PLP

11.9.1 Neuromodulation

The search for effective treatment thus continues. Neuromodulation in this context refers to the electrical stimulation of the peripheral or central nervous system, with the goal of relieving pain.

11.9.1.1 Peripheral Stimulation – Transcutaneous Electrical Nerve Stimulation

There are no clinical trials in the literature, which have examined the value of Transcutaneous Electrical Nerve Stimulation (TENS) for the treatment of PLP, but anecdotal evidence and the authors' clinical experience suggests that this simple, safe method of neuromodulation can be beneficial. Electrodes placed at truncated nerve endings at the stump can give projected paraesthesia into the phantom, covering the painful area and blocking messages at the "pain gate" in the spinal cord (Nnoaham and Kumbang 2007). However, many of the studies examined for this Cochrane Review were excluded because of poor methodology. Another limitation of TENS in this patient group is the occasional difficulty of combining electrode application at the site of the stump with prosthesis use. In addition, the efficacy of TENS is likely to wear off over time. However, TENS is inexpensive and safe and simple to use.

11.9.1.2 Central Stimulation

Neuromodulation in the central nervous system may be targeted at the spinal cord or the brain.

11.9.1.3 Spinal Cord Stimulation (SCS)

SCS has a similar goal to that of TENS, i.e., blocking pain transmission, but stimulation is applied directly to the spinal cord. This is achieved by the surgical implantation of an electrode into the epidural space, with a power pack connected and inserted into the abdominal wall (Mailis-Gagnon et al. 2004). The stimulator may then be programmed so that pleasant paraesthesia is felt in the area of pain, effectively blocking the pain messages, although the precise, complex mode of action of SCS is not known (Meyerson and Linderoth 2006). However, it has been shown to be effective for the management of severe neuropathic pain (Mailis-Gagnon et al. 2004). There are no clinical trials to show the effectiveness of SCS in PLP, but our own clinical experience suggests that, in carefully selected cases, when other therapies have failed, SCS may be an option. Patients need to be referred to a pain clinic, which has the expertise to manage this complex, invasive therapy.

11.9.1.4 Deep Brain Stimulation

There are some case reports of the beneficial effects of applying electrical stimulation to the thalamus (Bittar et al. 2005; Katayama et al. 2001) and the motor cortex (Katayama et al. 2001) with moderate benefit in a small number of patients. This is another invasive intervention requiring considerable neurosurgical expertise. It is still considered to be an experimental intervention. There is one documented case of a patient with phantom foot pain (within a larger case series), who benefitted from deep brain stimulation over a 6-year period (Hamani et al. 2006).

This review of interventions serves to confirm the fact that PLP continues to be a pain syndrome with no one treatment which is certain to give relief.

11.10 Psychological Factors Affecting Phantom Limb Pain

As in many other chronic pain syndromes, episodes of PLP may be influenced by psychological factors such as stress, anxiety and depression (Sherman et al. 1981). Furthermore, the intractable nature of the condition and low treatment success rate of PLP can deter all but the most persistent and self-reliant individuals to seek an explanation and adequate support for their pain. Previously, such people were referred to mental health professionals, giving the biased view of PLP having "emotional origins"; in the worst case, the pain may have been labelled as psychogenic in origin. Today, many patients are still unwilling to report the pain they are experiencing, in case they are told that it is "all in their head."

The loss of a limb is a major event with many psychological implications. Many PLP sufferers, like the general population of chronic pain suffers (who may or may not have a physiological origin for their pain), show elevated levels of fear, fatigue and insomnia, similar to those seen in people with depression. Reports suggest that anywhere between 20 and 60% of amputees may be clinically depressed (3–5 times that of the general population; (Ephraim et al. 2005; Hill 1999) and there is a well-known correlation between depth of depression/anxiety and increased pain levels. There is, however, no evidence to support the long-held assumption that amputees with PLP "somatise" their depression, nor are they "grieving" for the lost limb (psychosomatic factors are not the basis for PLP). Living with an untreatable chronic pain is very depressing for most chronic pain sufferers, including amputees, and PLP sufferers have normal psychological profiles for the chronic pain population (Sherman et al. 1981).

For many amputees, it is not the underlying condition (e.g., amputation of a limb) that primarily impairs the individual, but the chronic pain, which develops as a consequence of amputation. Amputees with chronic pain report significantly more performance difficulties and disability than persons without pain (Marshall et al. 1992) but not psychological distress or negative affect (Whyte and Niven 2001). In addition, over 50% of those with PLP report having residual limb pain (also known as stump pain), which impairs function and is negatively correlated with employment (Schoppen et al. 2001; Sherman and Sherman 1983; Whyte and Carroll 2002). Gallagher et al. (2001) report that amputees with residual limb pain experience greater levels of pain intensity and greater interference with daily activities than amputees with PLP. Stump problems are frequently painful and can prevent the use of prosthesis for extended periods of time, which may cause prolonged inactivity and depression for the individual (Williamson et al. 1994). For example, a study by Desmond and MacLachlan (2006) found that in an older population of traumatic lower limb amputees (ex-servicemen after at least 10 years post-amputation) depression was related to the amount of residual limb pain and was more a determinant of health-related quality of life, accounting for greater levels of pain-related impairment than PLP. It is not always apparent what is PLP and what is residual limb pain; residual limb pain is positively associated with PLP and they are commonly confused. For example, the stump or residual limb may also tingle, itch, cramp and have involuntary movements (Flor 2002). Stump pain is largely acute and can be treated with analgesics whereas PLP is neuropathic and does not respond as well.

Adaptation to limb amputation involves both physical and psychosocial challenges: disability, prosthesis use, change in employment status or occupation, changes in body image and self-concept can all act as stressors and trigger maladaptive reactions, poor coping strategies and psychological adjustment (Desmond and MacLachlan 2006). The outcomes and psychological factors affecting traumatic amputees (who are generally young, fit and healthy) will differ from those for disease-related amputees (who tend to be older and have more emotional distress and a poor prognosis). Limitations in activity, time since amputation and age have been shown to be significant predictors of poor psychological adjustment following loss of a limb (Kashani et al. 1983; Frank et al. 1984; Williamson 1998). For example, an elderly population is less likely to use a prosthesis, leading to a restriction of normal activities and the likelihood of depression.

Amputees with chronic pain may also experience altered body image and a balance between social networks, environment and coping mechanisms is needed to maintain and/or develop a positive body image after amputation (Ellis 2002). Psychological support in the form of emotional warmth and empathy, suitable explanations and advice, reassurance and hope and the opportunity to verbalise negative thoughts can increase trust in the practitioner and increased self-esteem in the patient.

The significant numbers of individuals reporting amputation-related pain (both PLP and residual limb pain), pain in the non-amputated limb and at sites taking extra mechanical burden (such as the lower back) indicate that pain assessment is as important as prosthesis care. Depression and anxiety should be treated as a priority. Psychological assessment, using a quick psychometric test such as the Hospital Anxiety and Depression Scale (HADS; Zigmond and Snaith 1983), combined with listening to the patient and observing behavioural clues such as tearfulness or withdrawing from social activities will help the clinician to evaluate the need for referral for psychological therapy.

11.11 Psychological and Cognitive Interventions for PLP

It is now well established that amputation is associated with neuroplastic changes in the sensory and motor cortices of the brain. More recently, these changes in cortical re-organisation have been linked to the prevalence of PLP. Therefore, many of the psychological and cognitive treatments currently available are based on providing efferent sensory feedback (in the visual, tactile, motor or thermal modalities) from the amputated limb to normalise the aberrant cortex. The treatments developed thus far can be roughly divided into two categories: (1) Treatments that apply tactile stimulation to the stump of the amputated limb in order to provide input to, and modify the cortex and decrease pain and (2) Treatments that seek to restore the image/function of the missing limb through virtual visual feedback from the intact limb or visuomotor imagery of the amputated limb and thus provide the motor system with the appropriate sensory corollary discharge from the limb to decrease pain.

11.11.1 Cortical Reorganisation and PLP

The cortical and sub-cortical systems contain two distinct neural maps – one for the recognition and processing of sensory input, and the other one for the delivery of motor commands (Kandel et al. 2000). Sensory and motor maps have an orderly, somatotopic arrangement of neural connections to represent each area of the body, but these maps are not fixed, and may change in response to internal or external challenge (reorganisation). Interest in this area began with the neurophysiological study of non-human primate cortex showing cortical reorganisation after limb amputation. The hand area invaded the face area of cortex after amputation/deafferentation of the finger digits (e.g., Merzenich et al. 1984; Pons et al. 1991). Since then, similar neuroplastic changes have been demonstrated in other areas of the cortex, for example, the utilisation of visual cortex by the somatosensory cortex in blind people for reading Braille (for a review see Sathian 2005). Animal work demonstrated how behaviourally relevant (not passive) stimulation of a body part leads to an expansion of the cortical representation zone (Jenkins et al. 1990), which prompted studies using direct tactile stimulation or a myoelectric prosthesis to decrease PLP via a reduction in the amount of cortical reorganisation after amputation (Flor et al. 2001; Lotze et al. 2001). For example, Flor et al. (2001) showed that after 2-weeks of training of tactile discrimination on the stump for 2-h/day, PLP had significantly decreased in correspondence with a significant reversal of the cortical representation of the limb as measured by neuroelectric source imaging.

Some of the best known behavioural evidence for cortical reorganisation has come from the work of Ramachandran and his colleagues (Ramachandran and Rogers-Ramachandran 1996; Ramachandran et al. 1992; for a review see Ramachandran and Hirstein 1998). He showed that some amputees with phantom limb sensations of the hand referred these sensations to the face such that, when the face was touched, stimulation was felt in the phantom hand (on anatomically corresponding digits). Furthermore, the tactile sensation was modality-specific (warm touch on the face felt warm on the hand). He also noted that a number of his patients could not move their phantom limbs, which had the subjective impression of being fixed in painful positions. This led to the hypothesis that PLP arises because of learned paralysis; the corollary discharge sent to the parietal lobes and cerebellum after a motor signal does not receive afferent sensory input to say the limb has moved and results in pain. To redress the incongruence between the sensory and motor systems, the motor system needs afferent sensory feedback to say the limb has moved. From this hypothesis, Ramachandran and Rogers-Ramachandran (1996) went on to develop the mirror box, one of the most well-known treatments for PLP.

11.11.2 Imagined and Virtual Visuo-Motor Feedback for Chronic Pain

In the mirror box manipulation, the missing afferent sensory feedback to the brain is provided by a mirror reflection of the intact hand, apparently situated in external space where the phantom limb is perceived. When the patient is asked to move their intact hand, their phantom hand is "seen" to move simultaneously in the mirror. In a sample of 9 PLP patients, 7 out of 9 felt their phantom move with this manipulation. A further four patients reported pain relief from spasms. However, the numbers in this initial study were small and the authors point out that such case studies are open to susceptibility and experimenter bias. They recommended that a larger, randomised controlled trial was required to test the efficacy of the mirror box treatment for PLP.

Despite continued interest in this potential treatment for PLP and, more recently, complex regional pain syndrome (CRPS) (McCabe et al. 2003), the therapeutic value of the mirror box has been based mainly on case studies and anecdotal data with mixed results (Moseley et al. 2008). Sumitani et al. (2008) found that a sample of 11 single limb amputees got some relief of deep pain with willed visuo-motor imagery after the mirror visual feedback procedure, but there was no control group. Brodie et al. (2007) found that mirror therapy was no better than motor imagery without a mirror. In one of the few randomised control trials of this technique,

Chan et al. (2007) found that 6 out of 6 participants had pain relief with the mirror box therapy (as did one of the controls) but the pain scale was not well-defined and the presence of bias was not discussed. In a single blind, randomised control trial on a larger population of CRPS Type I and PLP patients, Moseley (2006) found significant benefits of using a graded motor imagery paradigm (of which mirror movements were a part) on pain relief. Participants in this study spent 2 weeks performing limb laterality recognition (using photographs of hands); the next 2 weeks practicing imagining moving the injured/amputated hand and the final 2 weeks performing mirror movements vs. a control group who spent 6-weeks receiving standard medical and physiotherapy care. The results showed that decrease in pain correlated with improved laterality recognition and imagining the injured hand in non-painful postures during this graded motor imagery task compared to the control population. Pain levels remained low at a 6-month follow-up.

Taken together, the results of these studies suggest that mirror therapy seems to be no better than motor imagery alone (Brodie et al. 2007) but a programme of daily mirror therapy might be effective, (McCabe et al. 2003) particularly if part of a graded motor imagery programme (Moseley 2006).

The mirror box method links the visual and motor systems to generate movement in the missing limb but, as with the use of mirrors in all reflection-based work, the limb remains in a fixed spatial position. Similar in theory to the mirror box, but with the freedom to move the hand, immersive virtual reality has been used in a small trial ($N=3$) for PLP (Murray et al. 2007). Over a number of sessions, participants reported transferral of sensations into the muscles and joints of the phantom limb and decreased PLP during at least one session. Participants were able to relieve the cramping and pain and this was of most benefit to recent upper limb amputees. Again, however, because of the low numbers, the authors suggest this benefit could be due to distraction and a randomised controlled trial and greater numbers are needed to test the efficacy of this intervention.

In summary, virtual therapy might be good for those who find motor imagery difficult. The therapy may be a good rehabilitation technique to use because of the ability to simultaneously see and feel touch, which has been shown to improve tactile acuity in healthy controls (Kennett et al. 2001) and which may decrease pain in PLP, in a sense "virtually rubbing it better" (Moseley et al. 2008).

MacIver et al. (2008) used imagined movement of the phantom limb in a cohort of 13 upper limb amputees. Nine of the 13 gained significant (more than 50%) pain relief by learning to imagine purposeful movement of the missing limb several times a day. In addition, these researchers used functional Magnetic Resonance Imaging to demonstrate evidence of a cortical shift of activation patterns from the face area to the hand area (and vice versa) before the start of treatment, which was significantly reduced and related to pain reduction, at follow up. A large controlled trial will begin in the near future to further evaluate this technique.

In addition to distraction, sensory stimulation of the stump (using TENS, SCS, prosthesis, virtual reality) and visual illusions such as the mirror box, other manipulations aimed at decreasing PLP include those which fall under the general banner of complimentary alternative medicines (CAMs). Ketz (2008) in a study of young trauma amputees from military combat/training showed that many of them were self-treating their PLP often using CAMs such as exercise, self-management, biofeedback, relaxation and distraction. Other CAMs such as hypnosis, massage therapy, acupuncture and energy healing were used less but this is likely because they are not well known to patients or health practioners and need specialist healthcare providers to deliver them. Such therapies may be beneficial for many amputees but like many of the previous studies, these have been carried out on small numbers as case studies. Therapeutic touch (Leskowitz 2000), acupuncture (Bradbrook 2004), reflexology (Brown and Lido 2008) and applied thermal biofeedback to the stump (Harden et al. 2005) have all been shown to result in improved pain scores. The mechanism for pain reduction with these treatments, however, is not understood; there may be a sympathetic nervous system or psychoneuroimmunology explanation for their action or they may work via a secondary mechanism in that the patient feels in control and increases coping responses.

Similarly, hypnosis has been used in other painful conditions and on healthy controls to treat/reduce pain (e.g., Derbyshire et al. 2004; Derbyshire et al. 2008; Montgomery et al. 2000). Oakley et al. (2002) report 2 case studies where ipsative and motor-based hypnotic-induced imagery were successful in reducing PLP. The hypnotic suggestion was aimed at treating the phantom as a real limb and not treating the stump as the sole source of phantom pain sensation. Its action is similar to that of the mirror feedback mechanism (but without the encumbrance of the actual mirror or VR device) but may not be effective for all people, especially those who might need actual visual feedback for this mechanism to be effective or those who are not highly hypnotisable. For others, this may be a desirable option as the imagery can be recreated anywhere.

In summary, treatment strategies should consider the following; the age of the amputee (in relation to prosthesis); whether the amputation was due to trauma or disease; whether there is PLP, RLP or both; the quality of the pain (deep vs. superficial) and whether there is depression. In addition, large-scale randomised trials need to be conducted to provide evidence of the efficacy of the large number of therapies given to patients in an attempt to manage their phantom pain. Access to evidence-based treatment reduces the need for each individual patient to try several treatments over a long period of time, and is cost-effective.

11.11.3 PLP Treatment Plan

- Always begin with a thorough, consistent pain assessment. This should include basic psychological screening, checking what the patient understands about PLP, and what their expectations of treatment are. Refer for psychological therapy if there is evidence of severe psychological distress.
- Consider initial treatment with mental imagery or other available virtual therapy, such that the patient learns to use imagined or perceived movement to "think away the pain."

- Consider pharmacological therapy, either gabapentin/pregabalin or amitriptyline as first-line therapy. Consider the addition of a strong opiate if the pain is severe. Ensure the patient is aware of the limited likelihood of success. TENS may be used at this point, either alone or in addition to pharmacology.
- Refer on to pain clinic if these interventions are unsuccessful, where a trial of SCS may be offered.

References

Backonja M-M (2002) Use of anticonvulsants for treatment of neuropathic pain. Neurology 59:S14–S17

Bittar RG, Otero S, Carter H, Aziz TZ (2005) Deep brain stimulation for phantom limb pain. J Clin Neurosci 12:399–404

Bone M, Critchley P, Buggy DJ (2002) Gabapentin in post-amputation phantom limb pain: A randomised, double-blind, placebo-controlled, cross-over study. Reg Anesth Pain Med 27:481–486

Bradbrook D (2004) Acupuncture treatment of phantom limb pain and phantom limb sensation in amputees. Acupunct Med 22:93–97

British National Formulary (2008) http://www.bnf.org. Visited 02/02/2009

Brodie EE, Whyte A, Niven CA (2007) Analgesia through the looking-glass? A randomized controlled trial investigating the effect of viewing a "virtual" limb upon phantom limb pain, sensation and movement. Eur J Pain 11:428–436

Brown CA, Lido C (2008) Reflexology treatment for patients with lower limb amputations and phantom limb pain – an exploratory pilot study. Complement Ther Clin Pract 14:124–131

Chan BL, Witt R, Charrow AP et al (2007) Mirror therapy for phantom limb pain. N Engl J Med 357:2206–2207

Derbyshire SW, Whalley MG, Stenger VA, Oakley DA (2004) Cerebral activation during hypnotically induced and imagined pain. Neuroimage 23:392–401

Derbyshire SW, Whalley MG, Oakley DA (2008) Fibromyalgia pain and its modulation by hypnotic and non-hypnotic suggestion: An fMRI analysis. Eur J Pain Doi:10.1016/j.e.pain.2008.06.010

Desmond DM, MacLachlan M (2006) Affective distress and amputation-related pain among older men with long-term, traumatic limb amputations. J Pain Symptom Manage 31:362–368

Dworkin RH, O'Connor AB, Backonja M, Farrar JT, Finnerup NB, Jensen TS, Kalso EA, Loeser JT, Miaskowski C, Nurmikko TJ, Portenoy RK, Rive ASC, Stacey BR, Treede RD, Turk DC, Wallace MS (2007) Pharmacological management of neuropathic pain: Evidence-based recommendations. Pain 132:237–251

Ellis K (2002) A review of amputation, phantom pain and nursing responsibilities. Br J Nurs 11:155–163

Ephraim PL, Wegener ST, MacKenzie EJ, Dillingham TR, Pezzin LE (2005) Phantom pain, residual limb pain, and back pain in amputees: Results of a national survey. Arch Phys Med Rehabil 86:1910–1919

Flor H (2002) Phantom limb pain: Characteristics, causes and treatment. Lancet 1:181–189

Flor H, Denke C, Schaefer M, Grusser S (2001) Effect of sensory discrimination training on cortical reorganisation and phantom limb pain. Lancet 357:1763–1764

Frank RG, Kashani JH, Kashani SR, Wonderlich SA, Umlauf RL, Ashkanazi GS (1984) Psychological response to amputation as a function of age and time since amputation. Br J Psychiatry 144:493–497

Gallagher P, Allen D, MacLachlan M (2001) Phantom limb pain and residual limb pain following lower limb amputation: A descriptive analysis. Disabil Rehabil 23:522–530

Grond S, Radbruch L, Meuser T, Sabatowski R, Loick G, Lehmann KA (1999) Assessment and treatment of neuropathic cancer pain following WHO guidelines. Pain 79:15–20

Halbert J, Crotty M, Cameron ID (2002) Evidence for the optimal management of acute and chronic phantom pain: A systematic review. Clin J Pain 18:84–92
Hamani C, Schwalb JM, Rezai AR, Dostrovsky JO, Davis KD, Lozano AM (2006) Deep brain stimulation for chronic neuropathic pain: Long-term outcome and the incidence of insertional effect. Pain 125:188–196
Harden RN, Houle TT, Green S et al (2005) Biofeedback in the treatment of phantom limb pain: a time-series analysis. Appl Psychophysiol Biofeedback 30:83–93
Hill A (1999) Phantom limb pain: A review of the literature on attributes and potential mechanisms. J Pain Symptom Manage 17:125–142
Huse E, Larbig W, Flor H, Birbaumer N (2001) The effect of opioids on phantom limb pain and cortical reorganisation. Pain 90:47–55
Jenkins WM, Merzenich MM, Ochs MT, Allard T, Guic-Robles E (1990) Functional reorganization of primary somatosensory cortex in adult owl monkeys after behaviorally controlled tactile stimulation. J Neurophysiol 63:82–104
Kandel ER, Schwartz JH, Jessel TM (eds) (2000) Principles of neural science. McGraw-Hill, New York
Kashani JH, Frank RG, Kashani SR, Wonderlich SA, Reid JC (1983) Depression among amputees. J Clin Psychiatry 44:256–258
Katayama Y, Yamamoto T, Kobayashi K, Kasai M, Oshima H, Fukaya C (2001) Motor cortex stimulation for phantom limb pain: comprehensive therapy with spinal cord and thalamic stimulation. Stereotact Funct Surg 77:159–162
Kennett S, Taylor-Clarke M, Haggard P (2001) Noninformative vision improves the spatial resolution of touch in humans. Curr Biol 11:1188–1191
Ketz AK (2008) The experience of phantom limb pain in patients with combat-related traumatic amputations. Arch Phys Med Rehabil 89:1127–1132
Kooijman CM, Dijkstra PU, Geertzen JHB, Elzinga A, van der Schans CP (2000) Phantom pain and phantom sensations in upper limb amputees: An epidemiological study. Pain 87:33–41
Leskowitz ED (2000) Phantom limb pain treated with therapeutic touch: A case report. Arch Phys Med Rehabil 81:522–524
Lotze M, Flor H, Grodd W, Larbig W, Birbaumer N (2001) Phantom movements and pain. An fMRI study in upper limb amputees. Brain 124:2268–2277
MacIver K, Lloyd DM, Kelly S, Roberts N, Nurmikko T (2008) Phantom limb pain, cortical reorganisation and the therapeutic effect of mental imagery. Brain 31:2181–2191
Maier C, Dertwinkle R, Mansourian N, Hosbach I, Schwenkreis P, Senne I, Skipka G, Zenz M, Tegenthoff M (2003) Efficacy of NMDA-receptor antagonist memantime in patients with chronic phantom limb pain – results of a randomized double-blinded, placebo-controlled trial. Pain 103:277–283
Mailis-Gagnon A, Furlan AD, Sandoval JA, Taylor R (2004) Spinal cord stimulation for chronic pain (Cochrane Review). In: The Cochrane Library, Issue 3. John Wiley and Sons Ltd., Chichester, UK
Marshall M, Helmes E, Deathe AB (1992) A comparison of psychosocial functioning and personality in amputee and chronic pain populations. Clin J Pain 8:351–357
McCabe CS, Haigh RC, Ring EF, Halligan PW, Wall PD, Blake DR (2003) A controlled pilot study of the utility of mirror visual feedback in the treatment of complex regional pain syndrome (type 1). Rheumatology (Oxford) 42:97–101
McCarberg B, Stanos S (2008) Key assessment tools and treatment strategies for pain management. Pain Pract 8:423–432
Melzack R, Katz J (2006) Pain assessment in adult patients. In: McMahon SB, Koltzenburg M (eds) Textbook of pain, 5th edn. Elsevier Churchill Livingstone, London
Merzenich MM, Nelson RJ, Stryker MP, Cynader MS, Schoppmann A, Zook JM (1984) Somatosensory cortical map changes following digit amputation in adult monkeys. J Comp Neurol 224:591–605
Meyerson BA, Linderoth B (2006) Mode of action of spinal cord stimulation in neuropathic pain. J Pain Symptom Manage 31:S6–S12

Mishra S, Bhatnager S, Gupta D, Diwedi A (2008) Incidence and management of phantom limb pain according to World Health Organisation analgesic ladder in amputees of malignant origin. Am J Hosp Palliat Med 24:455–462
Montgomery GH, DuHamel KN, Redd WH (2000) A meta-analysis of hypnotically induced analgesia: how effective is hypnosis? Int J Clin Exp Hypn 48:138–153
Moseley GL (2006) Graded motor imagery for pathologic pain. Neurology 67:1–6
Moseley GL, Gallace A, Spence C (2008) Is mirror therapy all it is cracked up to be? Current evidence and future directions. Pain 138:7–10
Murray CD, Pettifer S, Howard T et al (2007) The treatment of phantom limb pain using immersive virtual reality: Three case studies. Disabil Rehabil 29:1465–1469
Nikolajsen L, Jensen TS (2001) Phantom limb pain. Br J Anaesth 87:107–116
Nikolajsen L, Jensen TS (2006) Phantom limb. In: McMahon SB, Koltzenburg M (eds) Textbook of pain, 5th edn. Elsevier Churchill Livingstone, London
Nnoaham KE, Kumbang J (2007) Transcutaneous electrical nerve stimulation (TENS) for chronic pain. Cochrane Database Syst Rev (3) Art No. D003222. DOI: 10.1002/14651858.CD003222.pub2
Oakley DA, Whitman LG, Halligan PW (2002) Hypnotic imagery as a treatment for phantom limb pain: two case reports and a review. Clin Rehabil 16:368–377
Pons TP, Garraghty PE, Ommaya AK, Kaas JH, Taub E, Mishkin M (1991) Massive cortical reorganization after sensory deafferentation in adult macaques. Science 252:1857–1860
Ramachandran VS, Hirstein W (1998) The perception of phantom limbs. The D.O. Hebb lecture. Brain 121(9):1603–1630
Ramachandran VS, Rogers-Ramachandran D (1996) Synaesthesia in phantom limbs induced with mirrors. Proc R Soc Lond B Biol Sci 263:377–386
Ramachandran VS, Rogers-Ramachandran D, Stewart M (1992) Perceptual correlates of massive cortical reorganization. Science 258:1159–1160
Robinson LR, Czerniecki JM, Ehde DM, Edwards WT, Judish DA, Goldberg ML, Campbell KM, Smith DG (2004) Trial of amitriptyline for relief of pain in amputees: Results of a randomised controlled study. Arch Phys Med Rehab 85:1–6
Saarto T, Wiffen PJ (2007) Antidepressants for neuropathic pain. Cochrane Database of Systematic Reviews, Issue 4. Art. No. CD005454. DOI: 10.1002/14651858.CD005454pub2
Sathian K (2005) Visual cortical activity during tactile perception in the sighted and the visually deprived. Dev Psychobiol 46:279–286
Schley MT, Wilms P, Toepfner S, Schaller HP, Schmelz M, Konrad CJ, Birbaumer N (2008) Painful and non-painful phantom and stump sensations in acute traumatic amputees. J Trauma Injury Infect Crit Care 65:858–864
Schoppen T, Boonstra A, Groothoff JW, Van SE, Goeken LN, Eisma WH (2001) Factors related to successful job reintegration of people with a lower limb amputation. Arch Phys Med Rehabil 82:1425–1431
Sherman RA, Sherman CJ (1983) Prevalence and characteristics of chronic phantom limb pain among American veterans: Results of a trial survey. Am J Phys Med 62:227–238
Sherman RA, Sherman CJ, Bruno GM (1981) Psychological factors influencing chronic phantom limb pain: An analysis of the literature. Pain 28:285–295
Sherman RA, Sherman CJ, Parker L (1984) Prevalence and characteristics of chronic phantom limb pain among American veterans: Results of a survey. Pain 18:83–95
Sumitani M, Miyauchi S, McCabe CS et al (2008) Mirror visual feedback alleviates deafferentation pain, depending on qualitative aspects of the pain: A preliminary report. Rheumatology (Oxford) 47:1038–1043
Whyte AS, Carroll LJ (2002) A preliminary examination of the relationship between employment, pain and disability in an amputee population. Disabil Rehabil 24:462–470
Whyte AS, Niven CA (2001) Psychological distress in amputees with phantom limb pain. J Pain Symptom Manage 22:938–946
Wiffen PJ, Collins S, McQuay HJ, Carroll D, Jadad A, Moore RA (2005) Anticonvulsant drugs for acute and chronic pain. Cochrane Database Syst Rev (3) Art No. CD001133. DOI: 10.1002/14651858.CD001133.pub2

Williamson GM (1998) The central role of restricted normal activities in adjustment to illness and disability: A model of depressed affect. Rehabil Psychol 43:327–347
Williamson GM, Schulz R, Bridges MW, Behan AM (1994) Social and psychological-factors in adjustment to limb amputation. J Soc Behav Pers 9:249–268
World Health Organisation (1996) WHO guidelines: Cancer pain relief, 2nd edn. World Health Organisation Geneva, Switzerland
Zigmond AS, Snaith RP (1983) The hospital anxiety and depression scale. Acta Psychiatr Scand 67:361–370

Chapter 12
Virtual Solutions to Phantom Problems: Using Immersive Virtual Reality to Treat Phantom Limb Pain

Craig Murray, Stephen Pettifer, Toby Howard, Emma Patchick, Fabrice Caillette, and Joanne Murray

Abstract Phantom limb pain (PLP) is a common consequence of amputation, and many persons with amputations experience vivid sensations of pain in the absent body part. PLP can persist for many years post-amputation and is very difficult to treat, since its aetiology is hard to determine. However, converging lines of evidence demonstrate that when visual feedback is manipulated appropriately to represent movement of an amputee's absent limb, it can evoke kinesthetic sensations of movement in that limb and decrease PLP. Most notably, the mirror box – where a mirror is placed vertically in front of the person with an amputation – is used in such a way as to reflect the image of an intact limb onto the phenomenal space of the absent or phantom limb. When amputees orient towards this mirror image kinaesthetic sensations can be evoked in the muscles and joints of their phantom limb, and PLP can be decreased.

Some researchers have highlighted limitations in the flexibility of the mirror box in providing a fully robust illusion of an absent limb as intact. Recently, three research groups have developed virtual reality systems informed by mirror-box work for the treatment of PLP. Although similar in intent and design, these systems have subtle differences. This chapter will outline these systems along with empirical findings, with a particular emphasis on the authors' own virtual reality system.

12.1 Introduction

Phantom limb pain (PLP), the chronic experience of pain in the residual impression of a limb which persists following amputation, can be considered to be one of the most distressing consequences of amputation (*see* chaps. 9–11 in this volume). Research has shown incidence rates as high as 85% with PLP sufficiently severe to require withdrawal from social or work environments for considerable periods of

---

C. Murray (✉)
School of Health and Medicine, Lancaster University, Lancaster, UK
e-mail: c.murray@lancaster.ac.uk

C. Murray (ed.), *Amputation, Prosthesis Use, and Phantom Limb Pain: An Interdisciplinary Perspective*, DOI 10.1007/978-0-387-87462-3_12,

time (Sherman et al. 1984). The relationship between PLP and psychological well-being is an intimate one. For instance, significant correlations have been observed between adjustment to amputation and pain, with adjustment to amputation less likely as levels of pain increase. The problem of PLP then is large and pervasive in the lives on many people with limb loss. However, while a range of pharmaceutical, surgical and psychological interventions are used to treat PLP, the success of these approaches is often limited and short-term (Katz 1992).

One promising avenue of research is the mirror-box, created by Ramachandran and Rogers-Ramachandran (1996) by placing a vertical mirror inside a cardboard box with the top removed, in which the person with an amputation places his or her remaining anatomical limb and views a reflection in the visual space occupied by their phantom limb (*see* Fig. 12.1). Participants were instructed to make various movements of their anatomical limb while focusing on the mirror's reflection and attempting to move their phantom limb in synchrony with the reflected image. Of five patients experiencing involuntary clenching spasms, four patients experienced relief through the mirror box. One patient experienced a gradual telescoping of the limb, which "amputated" the phantom elbow and, with it, the phantom pains he experienced in that elbow. The majority of patients experienced some form of transferred kinesthetic sensations into the muscles and joints of their phantom limb while using the equipment. According to Ramachandran, when a limb is intact, motor commands in the brain to move a limb are usually damped by error feedback, such as vision and from proprioception. With a phantom limb such damping is not

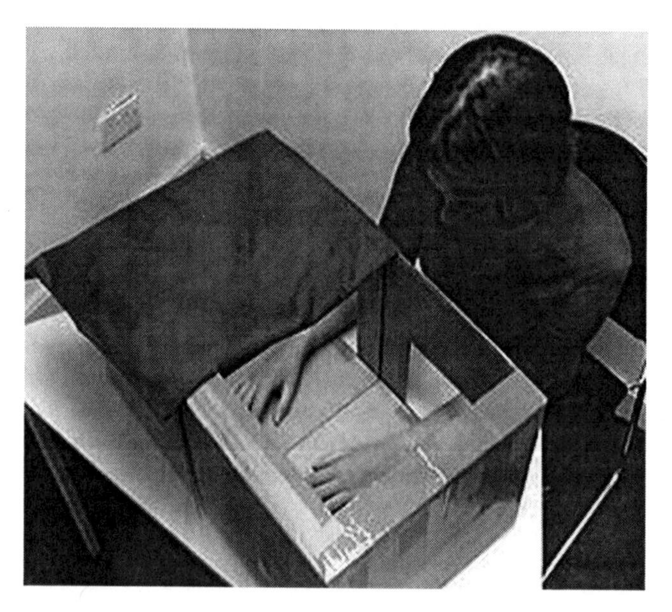

Fig. 12.1 The mirror box in use. Copyright Dublin Psychoprosthetics Group. Used with permission

possible and the motor output becomes amplified, which may then be experienced as painful.

The mirror-box has also been used with similar success with lower-limb amputees, where viewing a reflection of an anatomical limb in the phenomenal space of a phantom limb resulted in amputees reporting a significantly greater number of movements of their phantom limb than with attempted movement alone (Brodie et al. 2003). MacLachlan et al. (2004) have also presented a case study in which the mirror box reduced PLP in a lower-limb amputee.

Blakemore et al. (2002) explain the mirror box phenomenon in terms of a central nervous system internal forward model in which the body and its interaction with the world are represented. The forward model predicts the sensory consequences of motor commands whenever movements are made. This means that the normal experience of a limb is based upon a predicted rather than an actual state. In the absence of a limb motor commands are still made, so that if a prediction of movement is made then movement will be experienced in a phantom limb. However, because the limb does not actually move there is a discrepancy between these predicted and actual states. With time the forward models will adapt to this situation, so that movement is no longer experienced in a phantom even when motor commands to do so are issued.

Therefore, when the mirror-box is able to restore voluntary movement of a phantom limb, then it is because the forward models are updated. The efference copy produced in parallel with the motor commands generates changes in the predicted position of the amputated limb that matches what the person with an amputation sees in the mirror.

While the above work and theory indicates that the mirror box may be an effective treatment for painful and paralysed phantom limb experience, as yet there are no controlled studies which have explored the number and lengths of mirror-box sessions necessary to effect change, how long such change lasts for, which types of amputation and phantom limb phenomenology respond best, psychological variables which predict who will respond best to such therapy, and any potential negative responses to mirror box therapy. However, there is a general consensus in the research community that mirror-box therapy does work in a lot of cases (Phillips 2000; Ramachandran 2005; Rosen and Lundborg 2005; Sathian et al. 2000; Stevens and Phillips Stoykov 2003).

Despite the apparent promise of the mirror-box, it presents a number of inherent limitations in treating PLP, highlighted previously by the authors (Murray et al. 2005). The illusion is tentative, relying on the patient to maintain attentional focus on the reflected image as opposed to the moving anatomical limb. The mirror box operates within a narrow spatial dimension, requiring the patient to remain in a restricted, fixed position. In addition, the possible movements that can be induced in the phantom limb are often constrained by the need for patients to imagine themselves carrying out two-handed tasks that are concordant with synchronous mirror-image movement – conducting with both hands, for example. Mirror-box work sometimes uses two-handed tasks, or bimanual movements, so that the patient can focus on both limbs (intact and reflected). With single handed-tasks, it becomes more difficult for the patient to ignore the visual information coming from their intact limb.

Research and theory on the mirror-box suggest that other visual therapies that work in similar ways, but which surmount the inherent problems of mirror-based therapy, may also relieve PLP as well as increasing volitional movement in phantom limbs. This realisation has led to the recent proposal for the use of virtual reality technology to treat PLP.

Although not intended as a treatment for PLP, Kuttuva et al. (2003, 2005) developed a virtual environment that gives persons with upper-limb amputations a virtual hand that could manipulate objects within it (*see* Fig. 12.2). This system used myokinetic activity of the residual limb for the intentional control of virtual hand motions. Users were able to manipulate virtual objects such as balls and pegs in a 3D training environment presented to them on a computer monitor, while their performance at various difficulty levels was scored. In preliminary tests, participants

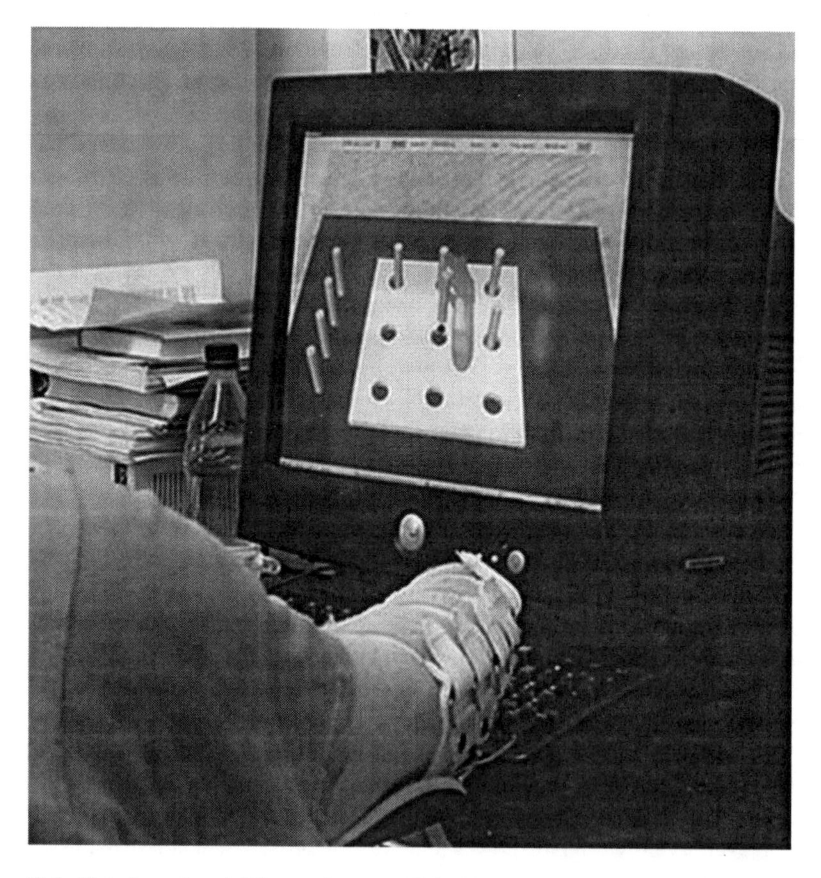

Fig. 12.2 Virtual peg-board filling task accomplished by an amputee wearing a sensing sleeve (Kuttuva et al. 2003). Copyright Rutgers Tele-Rehabilitation Institute (www.ti.rutgers.edu). Used with permission

were readily able to grasp and release virtual objects. These researchers proposed the utility of the system as an assessment tool for rehabilitation engineers, and as a motivator for those with limb loss to exercise and thereby maintain their residual motor ability. However, perhaps because these researchers specialised in disciplines like electrical, computer and biomedical engineering, they did not discuss in depth the potential of such work for the treatment of PLP.

Since the publication of this work, three research groups have developed similar virtual systems where the intention is to treat PLP. The rationales advanced by these VR advocates for why it might have efficacy beyond that offered by the simpler mirror box include the flexibility of the technology to manipulate and present representations of the body, including the phantom limb. In what follows we will present the development and exploratory findings of three virtual reality systems for the treatment of PLP: namely, an Augmented Virtual Reality system by the Dublin Psychoprosthetics Group (O'Neill et al. 2003; Desmond et al. 2006); a Virtual Agency system by Cole and Colleagues (Cole et al. 2009); and our own Immersive Virtual Reality system (Murray et al. 2005, 2006a, b, c, 2007). In the following sections, we will provide an overview of these, with particular emphasis on our own work.

12.2 Augmented Virtual Reality: The Dublin Psychoprosthetics Group

The Dublin Psychoprosthetics Group points out that there are methodological constraints inherent in the use of conventional mirrors, including the task symmetry in bimannual movement of anatomical and reflected limbs, the dependant nature of visual feedback on the movement of an intact limb and the lack of phenomenological correspondence between the intact anatomical limb and the often idiosyncratic topography of phantom limbs (namely, "irregularly shaped" phantoms) (O'Neill et al. 2003). They therefore sought to develop a system which would enable the control of a virtual phantom by the remaining corresponding anatomical limb, and which could potentially be adapted so that it produced a virtual representation tailored to the phenomenological experience of a phantom limb by the person using the system (*see* Fig. 12.3).

The solution they arrived at was an Augmented Reality system for unilateral upper-limb amputees (O'Neill et al. 2003; Desmond et al. 2006). This consisted of a three-dimensional (3D) graphical representation of an arm controlled by a wireless data glove (worn on the intact arm) and presented on a flat computer screen. The data glove allows for the measurement and representation of finger flexure and the orientation of the user's hand. As movements of the intact hand are made, the information received from the glove is translated into movements of the virtual facsimile in real time. Movements of the virtual facsimile are therefore controlled by movement of the data glove and appear to the user on a screen in an analogous fashion to the reflected limb in mirror-box work. Alternatively, the system enables

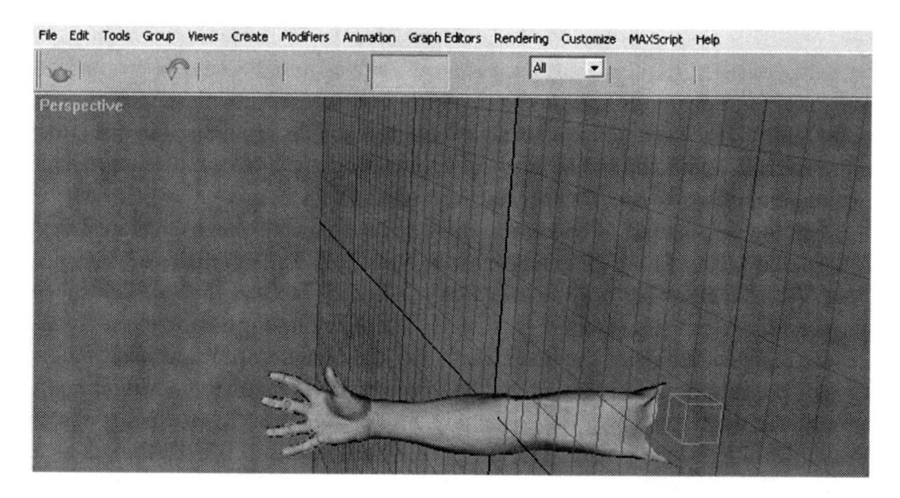

Fig. 12.3 Graphical representation of an arm in the Dublin Psychoprosthetics Group's Augmented Virtual Reality system that can be altered to represent the phantom limb as it is perceived to look by the person concerned. Originally published in O'Neill et al. (2003) Copyright Dublin Psychoprosthetics Group. Used with permission

the remote control of these virtual movements via a computer. The system includes a facility so that either bimanual symmetrical movements can be made, or that the phantom moves in the same direction of the animating anatomical limb.

12.2.1 Empirical Work with the Augmented Mirror Box

As with all the VR work on this topic to date, the Dublin Psychoprosthetics group has conducted exploratory empirical work to enable preliminary evaluation of the changes in phantom limb phenomenology afforded by their system (Desmond et al. 2006). Before allowing participants to use the system, the authors carried out semi-structured interviews describing amputation history, prosthesis use, and phantom limb experiences. Three participants were included in the study. The first participant was a 40-year-old man who used a passive prosthesis and who had undergone right-side transhumeral amputation because of osteogenic sarcoma, approximately 3 years before participating in the study. Participant 2 was a 25-year-old man whose amputation of the right forequarter was the result of a motor vehicle accident 6 years earlier. He also used a passive cosmetic prosthesis for social occasions only. Participant 3 was a 49-year-old woman who had an amputation of her right arm distal to the elbow following a motor vehicle accident, approximately 12 years earlier. She mainly wore a cosmetic prosthesis but also used a myoelectric prosthesis for particular tasks.

During the experimental phase of the study, participants wore a data glove on their intact arm and carried out a series of symmetric and asymmetric arm movements using both their phantom and contralateral arms. These movements required participants to hold their hands flat and simultaneously tap their index fingers, or to attempt movement of all fingers simultaneously while they held the palm of their hand first towards a mirror, and in the following trials a flat computer screen. The trials proceeded in an exploratory fashion, with task demands varying for each participant according to both the varying levels of volitional control participants had over their phantoms and their reactions to the visual feedback. The task demands were varied across participants to appropriately consider their individual experiences and reactions. Participants opted to wear their prostheses during the trial.

For two participants (P1 and P3) phantom limb experience was altered and intensified using either visual feedback via a standard mirror or via the augmented mirror, although for P1 this effect was more pronounced during the use of the standard mirror. When inconsistent feedback was presented (as in showing the image of the phantom as stationary when the participant was trying to move his phantom fingers) the phantom experience in particular fingers was reduced. In contrast, the presentation of inconsistent feedback in the standard mirror condition induced phantom pain. Although the reason for this discrepancy is unclear, the authors note that Participant 1 related how emotional stress could trigger phantom pain. The authors suggest how it was possible that at the end of the testing session, when the standard mirror was reintroduced, the participant might have been tired and frustrated by the task, therefore inducing pain (although he did not believe this to be the case himself). Viewing the augmented reality phantom image facilitated greater movement of the phantom index finger for Participant 3. Although such movement had previously been impossible, the virtual arm aided independent movement of her third and fourth fingers. Movement of the fingers of their phantom hand could also be remotely generated. In contrast, before testing, Participant 2 was unable to produce voluntary movement in his phantom, and use of either the standard mirror or the augmented reality box had no effect on the volitional control of his phantom.

In considering the unique contribution of their study, Desmond et al. (2006) highlight their observation that incongruent movement of the phantom limb, visually fed-back via the augmented reality box, may reduce the perception of discomfort and pain. They note that this observation had not previously been possible without augmented reality technology. For Participant 1, attempts to move his phantom while viewing an image of a partially frozen hand (where some but not all of the visually presented fingers were free to move in tandem with the movement of the data glove) resulted in the alleviation of discomfort in the seemingly frozen fingers. This finding contrasts with a later observation in the same participant that incongruent feedback provided by the conventional mirror induced phantom pain, which the authors suggested warranted additional study.

When Participant 3's virtual facsimile was controlled remotely, she felt her phantom fingers move in tandem with the externally controlled phantom image. The authors argue that this finding has potential clinical utility, suggesting that exposure to visual cues may help to free painfully clenched or positioned phantoms. However, they cite as a note of caution a study by Giraux and Sirigu (2003), who observed that passively exposing individuals with brachial plexus avulsion to prerecorded arm movements could also induce painful phantom experiences.

Desmond et al. (2006) highlight that while their exploratory study focused on feedback of noncontingent phantom limb movement, their system allows for a stronger test of the hypothesis that visual feedback of a "virtual arm" increases awareness and/or controllability of a phantom limb and reduces phantom pain. This could be achieved by using limb representations that incorporate postures and structures particular to individuals' phantoms but not readily reproducible using conventional mirrors. However, the ability to present phenomenologically accurate representations of phantom limbs is a potential property of all VR systems discussed here. How changes in the virtual representation could be modified over time to best facilitate PLP relief is an interesting issue, but not discussed in depth by the authors.

12.3 Virtual Agency: Cole and Colleagues

In contrast to the Dublin Psychoprosthetics Group (and our own system to be discussed later), where a contralateral anatomical limb is used to animate a virtual limb in the phenomenological space of a phantom limb, Cole and colleagues developed a virtual system in which the remaining portion of an amputated upper or lower limb was used to control an intact virtual limb representation. This is similar to the system developed by Kuttuva et al. (2005), discussed earlier. The aim is to make the participants gain agency for the virtually presented limb, which the authors hypothesized would reduce PLP. The proposed advantages of the system outlined by Cole and colleagues is that bilateral movements are not required, and that the movement of the virtual limb is driven by movement on the same side of the participant's body (and the correct side of the brain). In contrast to capturing finger movements of the opposite hand, as with a Data glove in the Dublin Psychoprosthetics Group's system, finger movements are pre-animated.

12.3.1 Empirical Work with the Virtual Agency System

In order to gain exploratory data of the system in use, Cole and colleagues used a sample of participants with unilateral upper-limb ($n=7$) and lower-limb ($n=7$) amputations, in which motion captured from their stump was translated into movements of a virtual limb within the VR environment. Measures of pain in the phantom limb were elicited from patients before and during this exercise as they attempted to gain agency for the movement they saw, and to embody the limb. After this each participant was interviewed about their experiences.

The trials were run in a low light environment to facilitate participants' focus on the virtual display. Session times typically lasted 60 – 90 min, varying according to patients' levels of fatigue. Two virtual environments were presented using a standard computer and a motion capture device. Electro-magnetic sensors were attached to either the residual arm or the leg of the user so that movements of the stump were translated into movements of the virtual limb. Before starting a goal directed activity, participants performed a series of physical actions with their stump so that the gesture based system could be calibrated. Following this, movements of the stump were interpreted as physical expressions of a modeled gesture and determined probabilistically.

The first environment interpreted motion for a missing arm (*see* Fig. 12.4). Patients were required to grasp an apple resting upon a table. The achievement of this goal comprised a number of actions; namely to reach, grasp, retrieve and replace the apple. In the second environment, for participants with a lower limb amputation, the user saw a bass drum as they might view it while sitting on a chair. Here, participants were required to complete four goal-related actions; raising the leg, performing a forward, pressing action of the foot on the pedal, releasing the pedal, and returning to a rest position. The system developed to interpret the movements of physical performance was dynamically recalibrated so that it was responsive to changes in physical performance.

Participants, recruited through consultants in pain and prosthetics, were told that the project was experimental, that if there was any effect on their pain it was likely to be short-term and that, though a reduction in PLP was hoped for, the reverse could occur. The group with lower-limb amputations were aged from 27 to 72 (mean 49) years old, while the upper-limb group were aged between 36 and 82 (mean 56 years) years old. They were taking, or had taken, a variety of analgesics,

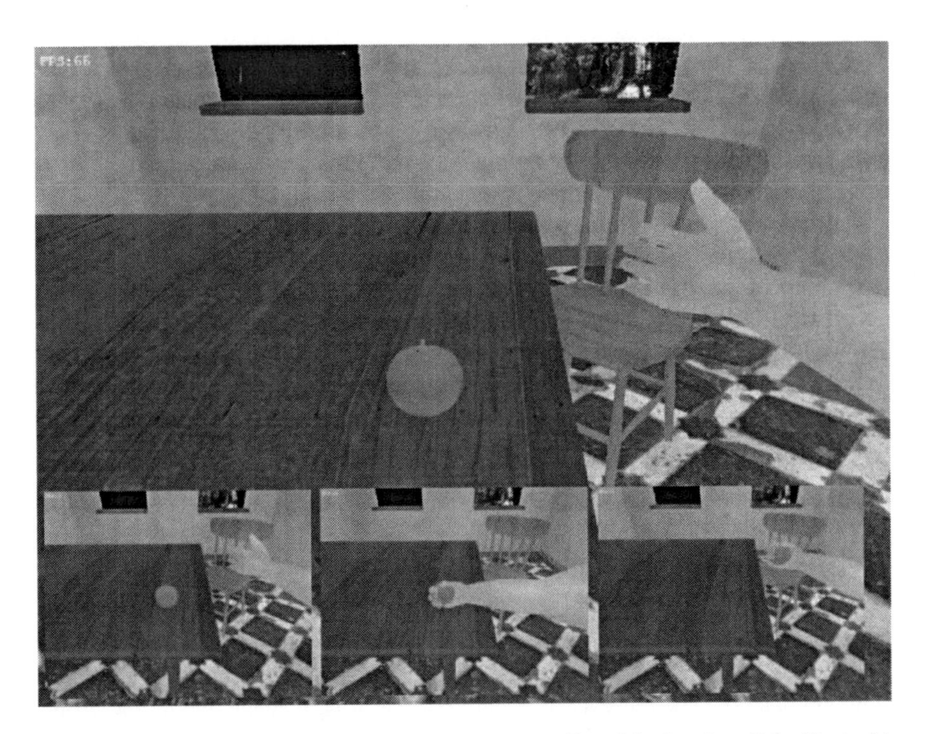

Fig. 12.4 Cole and colleagues' virtual arm environment. Copyright Jonathan Cole. Used with permission

and some had also tried acupuncture, hypnosis, and Cognitive Behavioural Therapy (CBT) pain management.

Of the seven participants with upper-limb amputations, Cole and colleagues report that five of them gained a sense of agency for the virtual arm, and did so usually within half an hour. Along with this sense of agency, participants described distinct perceptions. One man, with severe PLP in some of his fingers and elbow reported a "buzzing" feeling in his first two fingers as he controlled the virtual arm to make a grasping movement. Another felt touch sensation when picking up the apple, so that he experienced sensations not just of movement but of exteroceptive touch also. With the merger of an experienced sense of virtual agency and sensation, pain reduced. One participant remarked, "Now, when I move the fingers there is still pressure but there is no pain, they are not being ripped off or squashed," while another stated, "When I move and feel the arm, it does not tingle; pain disappears into the background and merges into the movement sensation." A third participant developed such agency following the trial so that her experience of her fingers in a painful clawed position changed to one in which they began to open and the associated pain reduced. Moreover, this pain reduction was of a larger magnitude than she had previously experienced with use of a mirror box.

Of the seven participants with lower limb amputations, four experienced significant reductions in pain. These experiences ranged from gaining control over the virtual leg to stronger phenomenological changes in the physical location, orientation of, and touch by the phantom limb. For example, one participant commented "I can feel the movement in the missing leg and maybe feel touch too. Once I am on the pedal I relax and feel my foot coming off it. It is second nature as though moving my full leg. The prosthesis is always a prosthesis; this is different. Here I am moving the foot. And at the moment the toes have sensation and though there is slight cramping in the toes there is no pain" (Cole et al. 2009, p 5).

Participants related how they "forgot" about or did not realise that their pain had ebbed away during the task: "Until you mentioned it I had not realised it was gone. One minute it was there and then, concentrating on the task, I did not realise it was gone," while another said that being in the virtual environment "lightens the pain" and went on to state about the virtual arm "I know it is not my leg and yet it feels as though it is." Once he stopped moving the pain returned "within a second or two, but equally when I move and feel it is me, the pain reduces." Another participant felt the touch of the drum pedal on his phantom foot.

12.4 Immersive Virtual Reality: Murray and Colleagues

Our own system is informed by the principles of mirror-box work in a way similar to that of the Dublin Psychprosthetics Group. The crucial difference to both Cole and Dublin's systems, however, is the immersion of participants within the virtual environment, rather than making them look at a screen, so that they feel present and embodied within the virtual scene. A head-mounted display (HMD) is used to present the computer-generated environments to participants and to facilitate immersion. In order to monitor and represent participants' anatomical movements data glove and sensors are used for those with upper-limb amputations, while sensors are used for lower-limb amputees. Sensors are attached to the shoulder, elbow and wrist joints or the thigh, knee and ankle joints for upper- and lower-limb amputees, respectively. A Polhemus Fastrak monitors head movements and arm/leg movements.

This system provides a visual representation of the whole body (as it would be seen from an embodied point of view) and uses algorithms in the software to transpose the movements made by the intact anatomical limb into movements of a virtual limb in the phenomenal space occupied by the phantom limb. Transferring a movement from a limb to another is possible due to the joint angles parameterization. For example, once the joint angles are recovered from the right arm through inverse kinematics, applying these joint angles to the left arm results in mirroring the movement. This method of transferral as well as other implemented software generates responsive, fluent, real-time motion, allowing virtual limbs to move in synchrony with anatomical limbs.

The use of IVR overcomes some of the drawbacks of the mirror-box, allowing the patient to perform tasks without having to remain visually and spatially fixed with a relatively narrow dimension. Furthermore, our use of IVR affords unrestricted movement within the virtual environment (VE). The participant could, if they wished, turn 360°. These actions would not compromise the illusion afforded by the system (i.e., the transposition of movements made by an anatomical limb into movements by a virtual limb in the phenomenal space of the phantom limb, as it would in mirror-box work). The tasks that can be implemented in IVR can therefore be more complex, and involve a wider range of anatomical movements than is possible with the mirror-box. A further advantage is the ability of an IVR system to implement single-handed tasks, and the potential to implement tasks similar to those used in normal physical rehabilitation contexts.

A minimal virtual environment (VE) represents the participant within a room, from an embodied point of view (*see* Figs. 12.5 and 12.6). Participants are provided with a number of tasks in this virtual environment in order to provide opportunities for hand–eye and foot–eye coordination of their virtual limb. These tasks are similar to the physical therapy and functional rehabilitation exercises previously used in desk-top implementations of VEs (Popescu et al. 2000) and are described below.

While the system gives realistic results at a gross level, there are certain constraints imposed on the level of detail at which the virtual limb can be presented. For example, features such as fingernails, fine joint creases and muscle tone are omitted from the virtual body (*see* Fig. 12.6). Experiments such as the Rubber Hand Illusion (Botvinik and Cohen 1998) show how an alien object, such as a rubber glove, can be incorporated into the body image in the absence of visual feedback from an actual limb. The success of this illusion seems to be that the tactile stimulus to the glove is applied in perfect synchrony with the tactile stimulation to the hand, rather than the glove looking at all human-like. This is especially the case when non-corporeal objects are used as extensions of the body, such as tables and chairs. These experiments lead us to infer that real-time response of the virtual

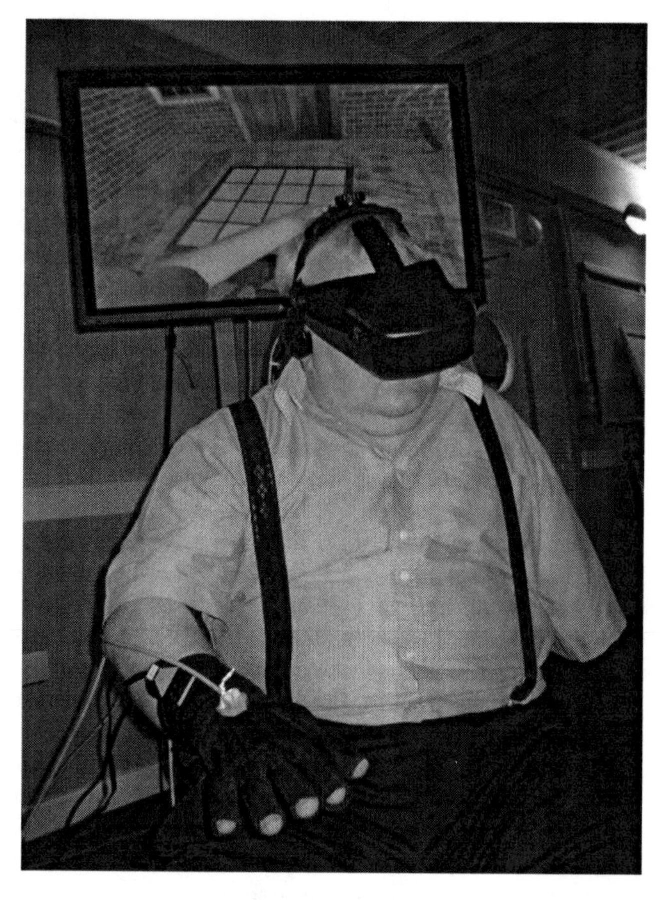

Fig. 12.5 Murray and colleagues' system in use. Copyright the Advanced Interfaces Group, University of Manchester. Used with Permission

limbs is more important than exact replication of the limb. Hence, the sacrifice of this fine-level detail in the virtual limb was deemed worthwhile to allow responsive, fluent motion. However, in an attempt to reduce discrepancy, the interface on start-up does allow the colour of skin and clothes to be altered to approximate those of the participant. It also has an option to include shadows to increase realism.

12.4.1 Empirical Work with the Immersive Virtual Reality System

To date the empirical work using our system has largely been exploratory, involving a small group of participants and examining qualitatively their phenomenological experience during and following the use of the system. Participants were recruited

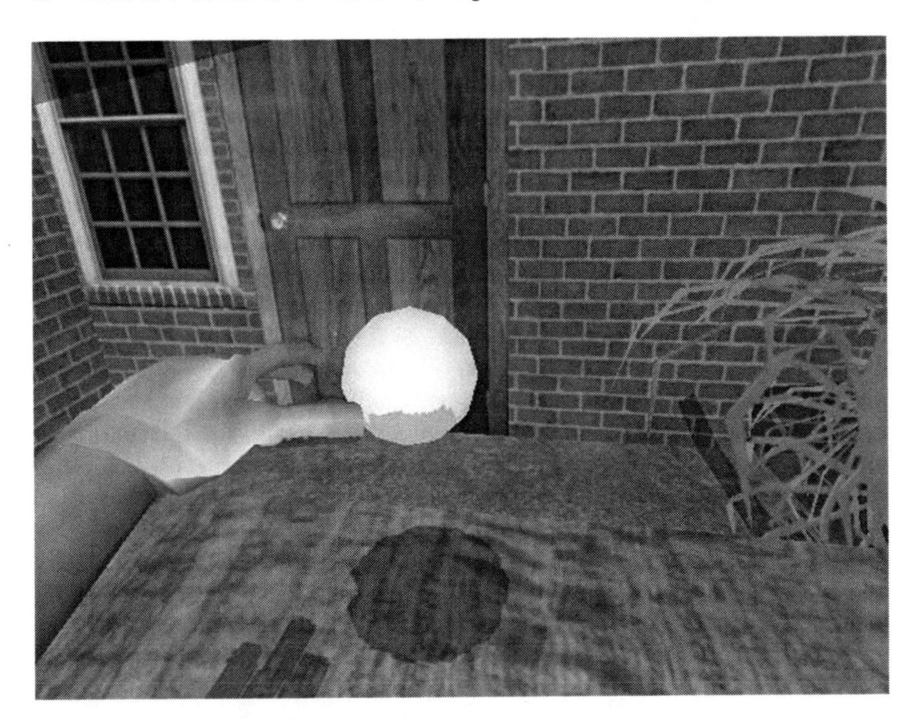

Fig. 12.6 An example of what participants see when using the system. Copyright the Advanced Interfaces Group, University of Manchester. Used with Permission

through clinical services on the basis of a number of criteria: having PLP; and being adults without any major visual or cognitive deficits. For upper-limb recruitment, only those with left-arm amputations could be included because the equipment (a right-handed glove) was suitable only for those with a remaining anatomical right arm. Participants with either left or right lower-limb amputations could be recruited. Participants were a minimum 12 months post-amputation to ensure the phantom pain experience was chronic in nature.

Eight participants were recruited after the inclusion criteria were exercised. Of these, three withdrew from the study after a maximum of three sessions. One participant was advised by his physiotherapist to withdraw his participation because of weakness in the anatomical limb used to animate the virtual one. The remaining two participants withdrew due to difficulties arising in transportation to and from the research site. Their ages ranged from 56 to 65 years, and their length of time since amputation from 1 to nearly 13 years. All participants had undergone varied and extensive previous treatments for their PLP; in the case of one (PK), this included the implantation of a deep brain stimulator, which had subsequently malfunctioned. Interestingly, 3 out of 5 had also been treated using the mirror-box with no success.

Participants used the system on a near-weekly basis, although the precise intervals between sessions were determined by participant availability and reliability in keeping appointments. However, all participants used the system at least 7 times, with a maximum of 10 sessions. At each session, participants used the IVR system for a period of 30 min, completing 4 tasks in repetition: placing the virtual representation of the phantom limb onto coloured tiles which light up in sequence; batting or kicking a virtual ball; tracking the motion of a moving virtual stimulus; and directing a virtual stimulus toward a target.

The small sample size precludes a meaningful quantitative analysis. Therefore we emphasize a qualitative understanding of patient's phantom limb experience, and of their experience of using the IVR system, in their own words. The broad approach here is a phenomenological one, with the aim of understanding patients' own embodied experiences (Murray 2004). Semi-structured interviews were carried out at each session (lasting about 15 min each), and participants were encouraged to speak aloud any part of their experience they wished to mention during the use of the system. Besides this qualitative data, Pain Diaries were also completed daily throughout the course of the intervention to allow a contextualised analysis of participant's phantom pain experience.

BH, a 56 year old male with amputation of the left arm below the elbow some 39 years and 8 months earlier, self-reported that his phantom pain, severe cramping in the phantom hand, "doesn't bother me regularly," but it was particularly stubborn in that it had persisted for almost 40 years. BH had very good voluntary control over his phantom limb before use of the system but reported highly unexpected sensations in the experience of his physical body while using the equipment: "It felt like I was leaning over to do it." He reported vivid sensations of feeling as though his right physical arm was leaning over his body towards the left hand side in order to make the virtual left, or phantom arm, move. This was a highly unexpected experience since his physical right arm would always remain on the right hand side of his body. It is highly unlikely that this self-report was due to confabulation since he continued to report this experience even after he knew that this was not possible: " I feel like I'm reaching right over but I can't possibly be because it's like a mirror so my arm should physically be going that way!" Interestingly, he also had a strong impression of his physical phantom arm moving while carrying out the tasks and found it difficult to accept the contrary: "it feels like I'm moving my left arm. But according to you, I'm not!"

In the last 3 weeks of involvement, BH reported no experience of PLP (previous reports and diaries had shown at least 2 episodes per week). While BH could not conclusively attribute this improvement to the use of the system, he did comment: "I'm not doing anything different from what I've always done… and I've not had the cramp since."

DT, a 65 year old female, had an amputation of the left arm below the elbow 1 year 3 months before taking part in the study. She had no volitional control over her phantom arm and her phantom pain was localized to the phantom hand. She described the pain in her fingers as, "almost as if they're trapped. My fingers are trapped. The knuckles hurt." The phantom hand remained paralysed in a fist: "The palm of my hand hurts, I think because it is as if they're [fingers] sticking into it." Her phantom pain was "there all the time" and often interrupted her sleep and everyday life.

DT reported vivid sensations of phantom limb movement during the tasks and, following the first session, that her index phantom finger had been somewhat freed: "It's funny… one of my fingers is coming out." She expressed extreme surprise at this new experience, "It's weird… I know that it can't be and your brain's telling you it is and you know damn well that the brain's wrong and it can't be! The brain's weird!" After the fourth session the phantom pain was reported to have eased overall: "the pain has gone down a bit and the [pain] flashes have gone down a bit… so it's been quite good for the last few days."

One negative aspect associated with DT's participation was that she usually experienced slightly more intense phantom pain for a period immediately after sessions. When asked how long this would tend to last, DT stated, "about 24 h. Yes, it spiked a lot and goes up but then it improves slowly." This verbal report was confirmed through observation of DT's pain diaries.

Despite the above negative aspect of DT's experience, the trend of improvement continued over the study period. By the final session both the phantom thumb and index finger had been released and DT reported having some voluntary control over these digits. DT surmised that this had a positive effect on the phantom pain in general: "I think the fact that it's brought my fingers out – at least some of them out – has helped the pain considerably. It feels more comfortable."

PK was a 63 year old male who had his left arm above elbow amputated 12 years and 10 months before the study. He experienced severe phantom pain "twenty-four seven. I'm never, ever out of pain." He experienced his pain as a "burning, cutting pain – like someone cutting me with a hot knife." He also had a vivid experience of a strap around his wrist that was "pulled really tight" and his hand was paralysed in a cup position with the fingers always being very painful. PK had little to no volitional control over movement in his phantom limb and could only swing it side to side with movement of the stump.

PK reported vivid sensations of a transferral of kinaesthetic sensations into his phantom limb while using the equipment which "allowed me to forget that my [phantom] arm was actually in a fixed position" and "it took away a lot of my phantom pain." After the 3rd session, the use of the system felt "more like reality than virtual reality." For the first few sessions, PK, like DT, reported increased levels of phantom pain after sessions. However, PK attributed this to the pain returning after a lull which increased subjective experience of the pain: "having had nothing [during sessions] and then having the pain, it feels stronger."

Following 4 weeks of using the system, PK was very surprised to report his phantom limb moving on its own accord for a period of 1 h while he was at home. During this time, he was "virtually pain free." Towards the end of his involvement PK reported, with some surprise, a number of changes in the phenomenal experience of his phantom limb which improved his phantom pain. The strap around his wrist had loosened: "before, the strap was so tight that my fingers felt swollen up and really, really painful. Now that strap seems to be not as tight, it feels as if I've got circulation." He could make very small volitional movements of his phantom fingers and had some control over the orientation of his wrist. Finally, he reported the experience of telescoping in his phantom arm which had a beneficial effect on the pain: "My limb actually seems shorter… I don't know why, it just seems to be shrinking."

SM, a 61 year old female with amputation of the right leg above the knee 11 years and 8 months earlier, experienced violent phantom pains on a regular basis which often left her: "passed the screaming stage… you end up crying." Her phantom pain at its worst was described as "electric shocks" which travelled down the leg and across her foot. This sensation would build up until, "as one if firing off, another one's following." She had good voluntary control over the movement of her phantom leg and foot and found that sometimes movement would "interrupt the pain."

SM reported a lowering of PLP during the IVR sessions: "It kind of diverts the mind away from the pain," and a transferral of sensations into her phantom leg throughout the tasks: "I was moving the limb itself and trying to get into the position you would actually use it – you know, to kick the ball." She also enjoyed the experience of using the system: "the right leg was trying to do it for me. I think it's a good exercise." However, her levels of PLP increased following sessions for a period of up to 48 h, which she attributed to the "stimulation of phantom nerves." Whilst SM enjoyed using the system and "exercising" her leg, in general her levels of PLP did not seem to alter much throughout the period of the study.

WW, a 60 year old male with amputation of the right leg below the knee 12 years and 3 months earlier, experienced intense pain in the sole of his phantom foot on a regular basis, "as if someone's ramming a knife in." He also reported experiencing many different kinds of pain in the phantom foot which he could attribute to previous pain experience in the right foot before amputation including: a broken ankle; a burn on the top of the foot, and even the memory of his toes being tightly squeezed when he was a child due to small shoes, among others.

The first session was terminated early as WW suffered with simulator sickness. During the second session his anatomical left leg collided with his stationary prosthetic leg which he commented was an "uneasy sensation… it looks on the thing [HMD] like it's not in the way but then you bang into it and it feels queer." WW also mentioned his phantom pain increased as a result, which is consistent with research that suggests sensory–motor incongruence as a possible source for painful sensations (McCabe et al. 2005). WW chose to remove his prosthesis during subsequent sessions to avoid this problem which helped him engage more, as well as report decreased feelings of nausea.

During sessions, WW reported vivid sensations of movement in his phantom leg: "It's a queer sensation… I'm doing the games with my right leg" and expressed pleasure at feeling as though he was "achieving" something with his phantom limb. After 3 sessions, WW used his experience of the IVR system to begin self-hypnosis; a technique, which he had once previously used to aid pain control. He would be "imagining myself on this machine and it seems to help a bit that I can look down and see my leg." It seemed that the virtual representation of the body helped WW to focus his concentration. He began self-hypnosis sessions 3 times a day using this technique; a factor which may confound the findings of this research.

WW reported that as a result of his use of the IVR system "the burning pain is abating a little bit. So it's improved a little bit." When reflecting on the experience at his final session, WW referred to an easing in the various different types of pain he experienced: "it seems to have taken the edge off them. You know, they're not as severe." However, WW's pain did appear to be the most inconsistent of all participants since he did not suffer with just one type of PLP; the pain would come and go at random intervals, making it difficult for him to comment on his pain over any extended period of time as it would fluctuate so greatly.

Although there is a need to be cautious in drawing conclusions regarding efficacy in case study reports where verbal reports are relied upon (*see* general discussion later), analysis of the qualitative data does provide opportunities for tentative conclusions to be proposed. All participants made some reference to a transferral of sensations into their phantom limbs during testing. This is a particularly interesting finding when we consider that three participants had paralysed phantom limbs, which could not be moved voluntarily. It may be, in fact, that this treatment would be most beneficial for those with paralysed phantom limbs as some phantom pain can be directly attributed to the inability to move paralysed phantoms into comfortable positions.

The reporting of sensations of movement in phantom limbs appeared to be more vivid for upper limb amputees. This finding could reflect the greater degree of movement afforded by the virtual hand and fingers as opposed to the virtual foot. Feet are less dexterous than hands, and this is a situation that is difficult to avoid in virtual reality systems. It would however, be possible to develop specific tasks using virtual lower limbs, which encourage the user to manipulate the foot in a more detailed way. For example, tasks could be made more difficult to force participants to use their feet in more dextrous ways. It would also be interesting to use a virtual representation of a foot, as opposed to a shoe, which may make the lower virtual limbs more analogous to the upper virtual limbs and reduce any discrepancy between the experiences of lower-limb and upper-limb amputees when using the system.

DT, the most recent member of a sample to have undergone an amputation (15 months previously), reported the most drastic change in phenomenological experience of her phantom limb. After the first session, changes in the once paralysed phantom limb began to help relieve aspects of her phantom pain experience, as recorded in qualitative reports. A speculative hypothesis could explain this in terms of a greater plasticity in the brain for more recent amputees as it has had less time to re-define the internal model of the body and to cortically reorganise, which is strongly correlated with PLP. As such, it is possible that this system may be of more benefit for more recent amputees. However, PK also reported significant experiential changes in his experience of his phantom limb after over 12 years of paralysis so this could suggest that the system is capable of aiding improvements in those with longer term PLP also.

Three participants experienced an increase in the level of phantom pain, which followed sessions. As PK pointed out, it may be that the easing in pain during sessions, that almost all participants commented on, means any subsequent pain feels more severe. All pain experiences are relative and subjective and a constant level of pain may be easier to overcome than fluctuating levels of pain, as is the case when pain levels were lowered during use of the system. It could also be that the increased concentration required to carry out the novel tasks actually have some temporarily detrimental effect on absolute phantom pain. This is an issue that would need to be closely monitored in future research.

As mentioned above, all participants did make reference to a decrease in experienced PLP while immersed in the virtual environment. This is a positive result, which should be investigated further. SM specifically used the word "distraction" when reporting this reduction, which suggests that at the least the tasks may provide a temporary escape from the phantom pain. It is important to carry out further testing, not only with a larger sample size, but with a control condition in order to assess any placebo affects of pain reduction caused by the novelty of the task. A suitable control condition for this research would be the use of the IVR system without any transposition of movement in the virtual world i.e., physical right leg movements would correspond to virtual right leg movements (Murray et al. 2005, 2006a).

One participant dropped out due to pre-existing weakness in his remaining anatomical, which meant that he found using the IVR system difficult. While the virtual tasks themselves were not judged to be particularly strenuous by this participant, the novelty of the tasks meant he was using his limbs in a way they were not used to. Obviously, it is crucial that use of this system does not exacerbate pain of any kind in any way. To ensure this is the case, it would be simple to introduce parameters, which control the difficulty and nature of the tasks to accommodate users of varying ability. A larger database of tasks would also provide the flexibility required when treating amputees of all ages and levels of health.

Finally, a crucial factor to be addressed in future research would be the intensity of the intervention. Previous work with the mirror-box has used regular intervention sessions of up to twice daily (Ramachandran and Rogers-Ramachandran 1996; MacLachlan et al. 2004). In the research reported here, participants came for sessions on a weekly basis which may be insufficient to facilitate change. This is understandable given that the majority of participants had suffered with phantom pain for over 11 years; it may be unrealistic to expect a weekly intervention for less than 3 months to have any dramatic effect on phantom pain. This is especially the case with this kind of intervention, which is not only novel for participants to get used to but also novel in terms of how IVR has been used in rehabilitation in general.

12.5 Summary and Discussion

In this chapter, we have presented work on the use of virtual reality as a potential treatment for PLP. We have described how this work has emerged from studies of the use of mirrors, which provide the visual illusion of a limb being present in the spatial position of an amputated limb, and one which is still experienced as a painful or paralysed phantom limb following amputation.

The three virtual systems discussed in depth here have a number of similarities, but also significant differences, and at present it is not known if any of these is ultimately more efficacious than another. They are similar in that all attempt to provide the illusion of seeing a limb, which the participant with an amputation accepts as a powerful representation of their phantom limb, and come to experience increased volitional control and pain relief in this. While Cole's system uses participants' residual limb or stump to control the virtual limb, both Dublin's and our own system transpose movements of the contralateral limb in an analogous manner to that achieved in the mirror box. However, while Dublin's group uses a flat screen in place of a mirror, our system is immersive: participants do not see "outside" the environment and willed movements of a physical limb are experienced as carried out by the opposite limb within the virtual environment.

The work arising from these systems is so far exploratory, and the different number of participants, inclusion and exclusion criteria, and frequency of use of the systems between the studies from this work, along with the largely qualitative evaluations of outcomes, not only makes comparisons between the systems difficult but also means that at present there is not enough data to give an unequivocal evaluation on the efficacy of such work. Controlled studies to explore the number and length of virtual sessions necessary to effect change, how long such change lasts for, which types of amputation and phantom limb phenomenology respond best, and which psychological variables predict who will respond best to such therapy, along with any potential negative responses to virtual therapy are needed.

Such rigorous work is required in order to be sure that there is a reliable effect at all. For example, one possible objection to the analgesic effects reported in the work arising from these systems is that such effects might be due to demand characteristics or a placebo effect (though Cole et al. 2009 collected quantitative data, which they suggest indicates improvement beyond that expected when participants are responding in a way suggestive of such influences). Randomised controlled trials with a larger sample size would be crucial to assess the efficacy of either VR system in treating PLP, not only over and above any placebo effects but also in order to extrapolate to the wider population of persons with PLP.

In this respect it is important to note that although the mirror-box phenomenon was first reported on nearly 15 years ago, there is little research that has put its frequently reported analgesic effect to the scrutiny of controlled studies (Moseley et al. 2008). However, given the more transparent benefits of VR systems to the traditional mirror-box, these provide a promising basis for such statistically-based work to be carried out. For instance, we claim that unlike the mirror-box IVR allows participants to perform tasks without having to remain visually and spatially fixed with a relatively narrow dimension. It is apparent that if the patient were to move away from the mirror, or not to keep the mirror within visual range, the illusion would be compromised if not completely broken. The "traditional" mirror-*box* alludes to the narrow, restricted dimension in which the patient is restricted. IVR affords unrestricted movement and potentially travel within whatever virtual environment (VE) is implemented. The patient could, if they wished, turn 360° and move location within the VE with simple navigational devices afforded by the hardware (e.g., the patient can use gestures of the hand to travel with the VE for instance). These actions would not compromise the illusion afforded by the system (i.e., the transposition of movements made by an anatomical limb into movements by a virtual limb in the phenomenal space of the phantom limb). The tasks which can be implemented in IVR could be more complex, and require a wider range of anatomical movements, than the mirror box. Again, this is transparently the case. For instance, in our IVR system the participant is able to bat away an approaching ball and watch it disappear in the distance. With the mirror-box they would have to wait to see a mirror image of the ball before they could attempt to bat it away (an almost impossible feat). A further advantage is the ability of an IVR system to implement single-handed tasks (mirror-box work sometimes uses two-handed tasks, or bimanual movements, so that the patient can focus on both limbs (intact and reflected). With single handed-tasks it becomes more difficult for the patient to ignore the visual information coming from their intact limb). However, in IVR, because the patient it totally immersed via a HMD, they have no visual awareness of their physical intact limb.

The authors of the alternative systems discussed herein also propose particular benefits of their own virtual implementations of the mirror-box. Cole et al. (2009) suggests that the control of a virtual limb by the residual limb is better in that not only is the correct side of the body being used, but the correct side of the brain also. In contrast, Dublin's and our own system requires agency to be directed towards the phantom limb when intentional movement is directed to the intact opposite which may increase task difficulty and make it more difficult to achieve the necessary agency to induce the desired illusion. Desmond et al. (2006) propose that the flexibility of VR enables the production of virtual facsimiles, which bear a closer topographical resemblance to participants' actual phantom limbs that may increase the illusion and resulting analgesic effect. At present, the implementation of this system is very similar to that of a traditional mirror-box (apart from the ability to induce movements in the phantom limb remotely and to prevent particular fingers of the representation moving even when the physical counterparts do). However, if implemented, the tailoring of phantom limb representations in this way would provide a significant line of inquiry not feasible with mirror-box work.

Clearly there are promising lines of research arising from these interrelated strands of research. While this work is suggestive of the potential for VR to provide effective relief for phantom pain, much work remains to be done. However, in any case, we do not advance VR as a panacea for PLP, but rather as a treatment which could have therapeutic effect for a significant proportion of patients.

We contend that IVR will emerge as a central technology for treating many types of disorders where the power of visual imagery can be harnessed to induce sensations that are ordinarily not possible. If this system was developed and had proven effect on PLP, the process and cost-effectiveness of implementing such a treatment would be justified. Health service costs can be reduced as a decrease in PLP can have "knock-on" effects for other aspects of patients' lives, such as financial instability due to unemployment. However, further work is needed in order to determine if such technologies do indeed offer virtual solutions to phantom pain.

References

Blakemore SJ, Wolpert DA, Frith CD (2002) Abnormalities in the awareness of action. Trends Cognitive Sci 6:237–242

Botvinik M, Cohen J (1998) Rubber hands "feel" touch that eyes see. Nature 391(6669):756

Brodie EE, Whyte A, Waller B (2003) Increased motor control of a phantom leg in humans results from the visual feedback of a virtual leg. Neurosci Lett 341(2):167–169

Cole J, Crowle S, Austwick G, Henderson Slater D (2009) Exploratory findings with virtual reality for phantom limb pain; from stump motion to agency and analgesia. Disabil Rehabil 31(10):846–854

Desmond D, O'Neill K, De Paor A, McDarby G, MacLachlan M (2006) Augmenting the reality of phantom limbs: Three case studies using an augmented mirror-box procedure. J Prosthet Orthot 18(3):74–79

Giraux P, Sirigu A (2003) Illusory movements of the paralyzed limb restore motor cortex activity. NeuroImage 20:S107–S111

Katz J (1992) Psychophysiological contribution to phantom limbs. Can J Psychiatr 37:282–298

Kuttuva M, Flint JA, Burdea G, Phillips SLP, Craelius W (2003) VIA: A virtual interface for the arm of upper-limb amputees. Proc Second Int Workshop Virtual Rehabil:119–126

Kuttuva M, Flint JA, Burdea G, Phillips SL, Craelius W (2005) Manipulation practice for upper-limb amputees using virtual reality. Published by Rutgers University, NJ, USA. Presence 14(2):175–182

MacLachlan M, McDonald M, Waloch J (2004) Mirror treatment of lower limb phantom pain: A case study. Disabil Rehabil 26:901–904

McCabe CS, Haigh RC, Halligan P, Blake DR (2005) Simulating sensory-motor incongruence in health volunteers: Implications for a cortical model of pain. Rheumatology 44:509–516

Moseley GL, Gallace A, Spence C (2008) Is mirror therapy all it is cracked up to be? Current evidence and future directions. Pain 138:7–10

Murray CD (2004) An interpretative phenomenological analysis of the embodiment of artificial limbs. Disability and Rehabilitation 26(16):963–973

Murray CD, Pettifer S, Caillette F, Patchick E, Howard T (2005) Immersive virtual reality as a rehabilitative technology for phantom limb experience. University of Southern California, Los Angeles, CA, USA Proc Fourth Int Workshop Virtual Real:144–151

Murray CD, Patchick E, Pettifer S, Caillette F, Howard T (2006a) Immersive virtual reality as a rehabilitative technology for phantom limb experience: A protocol. Cyberpsychol Behav 9(2):167–170

Murray CD, Patchick E, Caillette F, Howard T, Pettifer S (2006b) Can immersive virtual reality reduce phantom limb pain? In: Westwood JD, Haluck RS, Hoffman HM, Mogel GT, Phillips R, Robb RA, Vosburgh KG (eds) Medicine meets virtual reality: Accelerating change in healthcare: Next medical toolkit. IOS Press, Amsterdam, pp 407–412

Murray CD, Patchick EL, Pettifer S, Howard T, Caillette F, Kulkarni J, Bamford C (2006c) Investigating the efficacy of a virtual mirror-box in treating phantom limb pain in a sample of chronic sufferers. Int J Disabil Hum Dev 5:227–234

Murray CD, Pettifer S, Howard T, Patchick EL, Caillette F, Kulkarni J, Bamford C (2007) The treatment of phantom limb pain using immersive virtual reality: Three case studies. Disabil Rehabil 29:1465–1469

O'Neill K, de Paor A, MacLachlan M, McDarby G (2003) An investigation into the performance of a virtual mirror-box for the treatment of phantom limb pain in amputees using augmented reality technology. In: Human-computer-interaction international 2003, conference proceedings. Lawrence Erlbaum Associates Inc., London

Phillips H (2000) They do it with mirrors – Who'd have thought that you could make the brain pay attention to a useless limb, or even exercise a phantom one, with only a mirror for help. New Sci 166:26–29

Popescu VG, Burdea GC, Bouzit M, Hentz VR (2000) A virtual-reality-based telerehabilitation system with force feedback. IEEE Transactions on Information Technology in Biomedicine 4(1):45–51

Ramachandran VS (2005) Plasticity and functional recovery in neurology. Clin Med 5(4):368–373
Ramachandran VS, Rogers-Ramachandran D (1996) Synaesthesia in phantom limbs induced with mirrors. Proc R Soc Lon, B Biol Sci 263:377–386
Rosen B, Lundborg G (2005) Training with a mirror in rehabilitation of the hand. Scand J Plast Reconstr Surg Hand Surg 39(2):104–108
Sathian K, Greenspan AI, Wolf SL (2000) Doing it with mirrors: A case study of a novel approach to rehabilitation. Neurorehabil Neural Repair 14(1):73–76
Sherman RA, Sherman CJ, Parker L (1984) Chronic phantom and stump pain among American veterans: results of a survey. Pain 18:83–89
Stevens JA, Phillips Stoykov ME (2003) Using motor imagery in the rehabilitation of hemiparesis. Arch Phys Med Rehabil 84:1090–1092

Index

R

LaVergne, TN USA
17 December 2009

167230LV00003B/13/P

9 780387 874616